IN THEIR HANDS

A FIGHT FOR LIFE AT ONE MINUTE OLD

IN THEIR HANDS

A FIGHT FOR LIFE AT ONE MINUTE OLD

Emma Innes

with

Jamie Innes

All proceeds from the sale of this book will go directly to Early Lives, the University College London Hospital's neonatal charity, in recognition of the unit's life-saving work

First published by Shakspeare Editorial, UK, February 2023

ISBN pbk 978-1-7397590-5-6
      ebk 978-1-7397590-6-3

Cover @calimackdesign

Typeset www.ShakspeareEditorial.org

For Sophie and George

Glossary

ECMO   extracorporeal membrane oxygenation (heart-lung bypass)

EEG   electroencephalography

GOSH   Great Ormond Street Hospital

ICU   intensive care unit

NG   nasogastric

NICU   neonatal intensive care unit

NTS   Neonatal Transfer Service

UCLH   University College London Hospital

Foreword

There's a certain way of being in the world, that comes from an experience of deep trauma. As I write this, I bite my lip, fingertips poised over the keyboard, typing, deleting, then typing again. I realise how difficult it is to put into words exactly how you feel after an experience like Emma and Jamie's; an experience like mine. Something is etched in one's being; there is a change; a sense of the world as you knew it being shaken and, with that, an irrevocable vulnerability. I know now that I will live with this feeling forever, a fact to which many who have witnessed tragedy will also attest. For once that gossamer divide between life and death has been so cruelly threatened, the notion that we have any genuine control over how our life unfolds becomes a fallacy. It was always a fallacy. But now one cannot avoid the fact.

But - and the 'but' is the point of this book - we are the survivors; we are the lucky ones.

Throughout Emma and Jamie's visceral narrative in *In Their Hands*, you feel every moment of the horror of Sophie's birth. Emma shines a critical lens on the glamorisation of natural delivery, of denying intervention, that today is so often celebrated in popular culture. This pedestaled earth-mother image so far removed from the sad, yet inevitable, reality that *sometimes* things don't go well. It is paramount to share the message that a medicalised delivery is not a failure; that what matters most is a thriving mother and baby.

Happily, this story is one of hope, of love and wonder. It is a lesson to treasure the everyday, to celebrate the ordinary, to watch your children laugh, watch them sleep, breathe them in, absorb them in all their deliciousness, knowing how truly fortunate we are to have them with us at all. It is also a celebration of just how lucky we are to live in a country which, while under huge financial and social pressures, still has a wonderful NHS, with brilliant staff who, quite literally, put their lives into saving ours. I feel every ounce of the emotion Emma and Jamie have poured into the telling of Sophie's story, and the power of their dual perspective on birth, juxtaposing the feminine and the masculine, is both unusual and touching.

There is a unique bond in shared anguish. Emma and I met in University College London Hospital's neonatal intensive care when Emma's daughter, Sophie, and my son, Finn, were being treated there as newborns. The moments between Emma and me in Room One (the room reserved for the sickest babies) were fleeting— we were fellow sufferers in the foreign and devastating landscape that is the NICU.

When Sophie was well enough to leave intensive care, I wasn't on the ward. I entered Room One with the familiar rising panic— the desperation to make the ward round on time, to see my baby's stats, to wash my hands … only to find our friends gone, Sophie's corner empty.

She had finally recovered sufficient strength to move along the corridor to high dependency. I felt bereft. But, true to Emma's generous nature, she had left a card by Finn's medical notes. How kind, I thought, to think to write to me as you left! You had enough to contend with. I don't think I messaged you – perhaps you wouldn't have either? – but our fateful, chance meeting months later, on a sunny June afternoon, with our babies, well, that was absolutely meant to be and it's one of my happiest memories. I am so grateful we have been able to share our parenting journeys; that we've been able to revel in the magnificence of our truly beautiful, bright and happy children who fought so very hard to be here.

Thank you for writing this wonderful book. I hope it has brought you peace. Thank you for holding a light for those parents who have sadly had to experience the NICU, for those who have lost babies and those who have seen our fragile babies' lives held in the hands of others. Thank you for showing the wonder of life when we move through our darkest times and for highlighting what it is to be truly human—fallible and raw. Thank you mostly, for being my friend.

Harriet Brennan
Finn's mother (and wonderfully, now also Dara's)

Part One
Crash Call

Chapter One

It's four in the morning and I've just given birth to my first child, a beautiful baby girl. The most perfect being I've ever set my eyes upon.

I've pictured the moment a million times: sharing adorable newborn photos with friends and family; calling the new grandparents to gush about how wonderful she is; lying in a hospital bed blissfully cuddling my baby; putting her in one of her tiny new outfits; welcoming smiling, flower-clutching visitors. That's how it's supposed to be. Because that's what happens when you have a baby, isn't it?

No. Unfortunately, it isn't. Not always.

What actually happens is that a doctor solemnly enters the delivery room and says: 'I'm afraid I can't predict a good outcome.'

The story starts a few hours earlier on February 8, 2016. I'm twenty-six, nine months pregnant with a deeply longed for baby and in early labour. I'm relaxed, happy and excited to meet the little girl I've been growing for nine months. I have drawers full of neatly folded baby clothes, a perfectly organised changing station and a stack of well-thumbed baby care books.

Having been on maternity leave for a month, I have long since run out of chores to do. I'm impatient and want to meet my baby. I'm ready to take the plunge into parenthood. I feel I've been teetering on the edge of that precipice for weeks. I want to get on with it.

Rose-tinted spectacles fully intact, I spend the day sleeping or bouncing absentmindedly on an exercise ball and wondering whether I can really be in labour. I've been having contractions all day and they're becoming gradually stronger and more frequent. But I can't believe the moment has really arrived. It is surreal, initially almost anticlimactic. I'm in labour and yet there I am, pottering casually around our flat as though it's a normal day. Until the evening, it is a normal day. I enjoy a lie in, watch some daytime TV, eat lunch. The fact that I'm having mild contractions all day has little impact.

During my pregnancy, I've attended all the NCT classes, read the hypnobirthing and natural birth books and written the perfect birth plan. I'm fully immersed in the romanticised vision of childbirth: all pregnancy yoga, water birth and then emerging from the Maternity Unit a few hours after the delivery, perfectly turned out. As though nothing has happened. My vision of childbirth is one picked up from glossy magazines. It's not real. This means I'm not scared. I'm respectful of the process but I'm not terrified.

The books I've read all tell stories of perfect home births and sell a narrative which de-medicalises the process. They suggest that in most cases medical intervention is entirely unnecessary, harmful even. I have bought into the ideology. It seems logical to me that most women, most of the time, should be able to give birth without medical intervention or assistance. After all, we are animals and all other animals seem to manage. Why should humans be any different?

So the schedule goes: stroll into the Maternity Department, have a straightforward natural delivery in the Birth Centre, then walk the short distance home a matter of hours later, pushing the baby in her new pram.

We know that birth comes with risk, pain and complexity. However, society and the NCT classes my husband, Jamie, and I attended have given us a fairly simplified view that giving birth is very safe and natural, and that Instagram moments are an inevitable payoff for a bit of pushing. We expect, like everyone else, to be in the majority of people for whom everything is fine. Now, we know better. We also know that, ultimately, giving birth is indeed still animalistic and brutal. We now understand that the idea of choice and agency during childbirth is an illusion. There is either a good outcome or a bad one. All one can do is hope for the former.

◊

By early evening the contractions are fairly frequent, and I've put the hospital bag by the front door. Jamie strolls in from work, and casually asks why it's there. Turns out, he didn't receive my messages telling him I'm in labour. That explains the lack of response ... I'm surprisingly relaxed about this because instinctively I know that the birth is still a way off.

Casually, Jamie begins making supper and I potter into the bathroom, fully expecting to settle down to a hearty meal. But when I sit on the loo, my waters burst so spectacularly that I scream. A tidal wave of fluid bursting out of me! Like vomiting, but from the wrong orifice. Jamie claims to hear them go 'bang' from the kitchen. Like a water balloon exploding. Being a practical kind of person, my first thought is: 'Thank God the floor in here is wipeable!'

Once we've cleaned up and Jamie has accepted his supper will have to wait, we grab the hospital bag and set off. We don't discuss whether it's the right time to go; I think we just know. In a state of blissful ignorance as to what is about to unfold, we stop in the stairwell to chat to some neighbours before walking through the cold February night to the hospital.

Me: Oh, hi Maddy! How are you?

Maddy: Fine thanks, and you?

Me: Well, erm, actually I'm in labour. We're just off to the hospital.

Maddy: Wow. Good luck! Can't wait to meet her.

Me: Thank you. See you soon!

It's all so normal. So normal that we do as we have for all previous appointments at the hospital – we walk there. It doesn't occur to me to do anything other than walk. We live so close that by the time we would have reached the car outside our building, and then walked from the parking space at the hospital, driving would have been more hassle. And, anyway, my proactive spirit wouldn't allow for such an indulgence.

Perhaps unsurprisingly, given my relaxed state and mode of transport, the midwife in Maternity Triage looks decidedly sceptical when I suggest that I might be in full-blown labour. She mutters something about sending me home, and about the ignorance of first-time mothers, before reluctantly agreeing to examine me.

She carries out her examination and admits that, to her surprise, I am four centimetres dilated and in established labour. I feel a twinge of pride that I'm so calm I have blindsided an experienced midwife; also, a hint of smugness that I was right – I *am* in labour. I'm not just whingeing or making an unnecessary fuss; I'm not going to be sent home to wait it out; I am going to be admitted right now.

Having taken the customary tour of the Maternity Department and been shown the Birth Centre with its pools, mood lighting and double beds, I fully expect to be sent in that direction. However, the midwife notices that rather than being clear, as they should be, my waters are 'straw coloured'. Light meconium staining, they say. No cause for concern. Very common in babies who are late (I am six days overdue). 'Just because her gut is mature. Perfectly normal for a mature gut to start passing the first stool, meconium, before delivery.' But, to be on the safe side, and because meconium in the waters can be a sign that a baby is in distress, I am taken directly to the labour ward.

Gone are the dreams of the perfect water birth. Instead, I find myself being shown to a brightly lit delivery room. To the casual observer, it is a place full of torture instruments, a highly medicalised environment which seems far away from the idealised setting for the natural birth I had been planning. There is a hospital bed in the middle of the room, a resuscitation table ready for the baby, should it be needed, wires and tubes emerging from the walls and a desk for the midwife.

Nonetheless, everyone is relaxed, the labour is progressing smoothly, and I accept what the midwives tell me to do. I am a good patient: trust the people looking after me completely, don't question them, just do as they say.

◊

Jamie

The simultaneous sounds of an overfull water balloon bursting, disgorging its contents, and my wife's surprised yelp heralded the moment we had all been waiting for. All the books, NCT courses, birth plans and general worrying had run their course. Now there was no denying it; the baby was coming.

The heightened state of alertness. Adrenaline. Butterflies in the stomach. Excitement. Fear. Uncertainty. Will everything be okay? Will Emma be alright? Will I fulfil my twenty-first century duty and be the perfect father ready to rub my wife's back and tell her what a good job she's doing or will I meet Emma's predictions and faint? After all, try as I might to be manly, I generally have a panic attack at the thought of going on a plane and am too scared to spend a night alone in our house.

A clear sense of purpose. Get the hospital bags. Get Emma to hospital. It was evening. The long dark of February was well entrenched. Our brightly lit flat felt warm and friendly. Everything was shipshape for our triumphant return, including the white wicker Moses basket at the end of our bed on its stand. Teddy bear guardians at the ready to salute their new charge when she was delivered to them. Well, at least until they were promptly removed to follow safe sleeping guidelines.

Emma was a few days overdue and had had classic first baby mild contractions for much of the day. I had headed to work as there didn't seem to be much of a rush, and indeed there was no need to panic. We are natural worriers and fretters, but neither of us – nor any one close to us – had ever really had any major medical issues. Statistically you're safe, and statistically you're never the wrong kind of statistic. We were obviously apprehensive about what was to come, but there were no premonitions.

The night air was pretty still. I remember the streets seeming quiet, but then it was usually relatively peaceful, for London, in Belsize Park. The white stucco buildings flanked the wide road and our route up the hill toward the hospital. It was only about a ten-minute walk, even with bump. I suppose part of me did wonder what would happen if the baby slid out en route, but I probably reasoned, if that did occur then at least most of the serious business would have been achieved.

We wobbled our way to the hospital. The Royal Free is a true concrete monstrosity, but at night the brutal slabs of grey give way to the dark, and the warm lights twinkling out give it more a feel of a welcoming hotel than a foreboding fortress of life and death. We went through the revolving doors of the main entrance, past the patients in wheelchairs smoking outside. Along the bright corridor. Lifts on the left. A well-trodden path in recent months. Pressed the button for the floor which houses the Maternity Ward. I don't remember what Emma and I said to each other. We must have made some small talk. I must have tried to make some mischievous jokes or observations, as I tend to do when situations start to get a bit stressful. Out of the lifts. Stainless steel sliding shut. Step one achieved: Get Emma to the Maternity Unit with baby still inside. Tick.

We were ushered into the triage room. Emma was lain on a bed. I think there was one other mother-to-be plus family. It seemed strangely quiet – not many people around. No resounding screams. That was a good start. The midwife seemed busy and fairly uninterested. Emma was still leaking rather a lot of fluid so we got our hands on some big mounds of absorbent pads. Birthing gold dust. I recommend stocking up if you don't want to risk your towels at home. We could see the slight staining in the fluid. A slight brackish-brown colour.

Emma was wonderful. She was calm but had that lovely, slightly sad, softness she rarely shows in everyday life, but which must have been revealed by her anticipation and fear. I could see it in her eyes, in the way she cast her head, a slight softening of her voice. We can both be fully grown up and child-like simultaneously, and

Emma is at her most beautiful when she is like this. When she is feeling slightly vulnerable.

The midwife assessed Emma. Curtains drawn. A charming procedure involving digits being inserted into orifices to assess dilation. Everything about childbirth seems to have more to do with country vets sticking their arms inside animals than with any glossy mummy magazine. God I am glad I'm not a woman – they have my respect but not my envy.

Most first-timers arrive too early and take a long time to get going and so are sent home until they are ready. Not us. We were on the final approach for landing. They consulted about the straw-coloured waters. Nothing to be concerned about. It was mild and the baby's heart rate was fine.

We went along the corridor to the labour ward, relieved to get our own room and our own midwife from start to finish. Might things have been different had they sent Emma straight for a C-section? We'll never know for sure, although it might have avoided some of the worst of what was to follow. The hospital was following the NICE guidelines for mild meconium staining in a low-risk pregnancy to the letter. The baby would be monitored, but statistically there was no need for further escalation.

Chapter Two

Emma

What follows is hazy in my mind. It's the middle of the night, I am high on hormones and gas and air, and I am experiencing natural labour for the first time. I'm beset by the sensation of surrealism that is to be at the heart of the entire experience. I'm admitted at eight or nine in the evening; the remaining hours of that long night are a blur. All the events I register might have happened within the course of half an hour but that can't have been the case.

I am completely caught up in the primitive forces that have taken over my body. Since the waters broke the labour has been progressing quickly. It is now a totally different experience to the mild contractions I was having earlier. The power of the process is extraordinary. I'm lost in what is going on in my body, observing it and yet feeling as if nothing is ever going to be in my control again.

I concentrate hard on breathing in the gas and air. Concentrating on using it correctly is a useful distraction. Focusing on breathing through the machine helps carry me through the contractions. The pain is incredible but survivable, because each contraction is short-lived and there's time to compose myself again between them. The intensity of the urge to push is unbelievable. I couldn't stop pushing if I tried. My body is working to its own rhythm. It knows what to do with no conscious thought from me.

I ask the midwife how much longer it will go on for. She suggests maybe a few hours. What I think is minutes later, I ask how much time has passed and am told two hours. I'm in another world. Normal, everyday things like time are irrelevant.

At some point during the night, when Jamie fears I am getting tired and low, he produces a card he has made to cheer me up. It contains messages of encouragement from our closest friends and family. It has PUSH written in huge, capital letters across the front. I think how sweet it is and we laugh together, reading the comments everyone has made. Jamie jokes that he laminated it to protect it from the bodily fluids he assumed the room would be awash with during the labour.

In the card, Jamie's best friend Bradley, who will be Sophie's godfather, has composed a poem to mark the event. It reads:

> There once was a girl called Em,
> Who was ready to burst at the hem.
> The baby was due,
> And all of us knew,
> That there would be birthing mayhem.
> But she really had nothing to fear,
> With her Johnian friends so near.
> It would all be a breeze,

11

With a push and a squeeze,
And the birth canal open and clear!
And after this difficult test,
A baby girl added to your nest.
Cute, lovely, sweet,
A real pleasure to meet,
All of you most highly blessed!

◊

The room is now dimly lit, Jamie is sitting in the corner by the window and the midwife is pottering around carrying out her duties. It's like a little nest separate from the world outside. I am totally absorbed in the process. Everything else is forgotten.

I'm lucky. I was admitted at the start of the night shift so I'll have one midwife looking after me all night. There are no shift changes. She's with me all of the time and I feel very well looked after. I've heard horror stories of women being left alone for hours in labour. This isn't my experience. I feel very well supported and safe.

I pace the room trying to get comfortable. Try to drink the sugary drinks everyone recommends for energy. They make my mouth feel fuzzy. All I want is cold water.

Jamie calmly reassures me through each wave of pain. I focus on what he is saying to avoid panicking and losing control. We are a good team. I couldn't endure each contraction without him. He's kind and supportive and loving and funny. He makes me feel safe and comforted. He's my link to normality in an abnormal situation. There's no one on Earth I'd rather have with me. There's something about Jamie. He can be very no-nonsense but in times like this he is so gentle and nurturing. I don't feel remotely self-conscious about him seeing me in this animal state. I just feel loved.

I know that the moment I panic it's game over; I'll be begging for an epidural. I have to stay calm. In control. Have to keep breathing. Keep listening to Jamie. I'm proud of myself for coping with just the gas and air.

The sweet, kind, calm midwife says that everything is 'textbook' ...

◊

Jamie and I have been married for nearly four years. He is a geography teacher and I am a journalist-turned-press officer. We met while we were reading geography at St John's College, Cambridge. I've always found him very funny and I think our relationship flourished because of my ability to laugh at his terrible – and usually slightly unacceptable – jokes. It's fitting that even in these circumstances he is cheering me up with naughty jokes. He tells me he intended to prepare for the birth by buying a plunger and waders ...

◊

In the middle of the night, it becomes apparent to everyone else in the room that the baby is struggling. The midwife has put a monitor on my stomach so she can constantly track the contractions and the baby's heart rate. The reading is concerning. The notes describe the CTG trace as 'suspicious'. The doctors review the

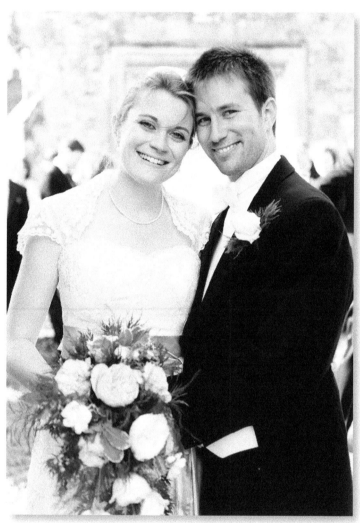

Jamie and Emma on their wedding day in 2012 (photo: Phoebe Landa)

trace. It's not sufficiently suspect for immediate action to be thought necessary and the labour continues uninterrupted.

The thinking is that she's just getting a little tired after a long labour. Her heart rate is having phases of looking concerning, but it's then recovering. The doctors consider this repeated recovery reassuring. It's believed that a baby who's in real trouble wouldn't keep showing these signs of recovery. She's doing a very good job of masking how unwell she is.

I have no awareness of the concern. I'm totally engrossed in what is happening inside my body. It feels to me as though the labour is proceeding naturally and effectively, so I'm satisfied. My body, while wracked with pain and intense urges to push, feels right. It feels like the right things are happening; it is at one with the process.

This begins to change when the doctors and midwives start to intervene. As they become more concerned by the CTG trace, and as delivery nears, they no longer allow me to stay in any position I'm comfortable in or let me walk around the room. In fact, it feels as if the process has stopped being mine and mine alone.

They tell me I have to lie on the bed with my legs in stirrups. I am uncomfortable like this. It doesn't feel right. I need to be able to move and I want to be left alone.

Earlier in the labour they had allowed me total control of the situation. They had looked after me and reassured me and given me and the baby the care and monitoring we needed, but they'd let the process be mine.

Now the mood has changed. It's become a medical emergency, not a natural process. Faces look serious, concentration written across them. A determination to deliver this baby as quickly as possible. They're kind and understanding toward me, but clear in their instructions.

I'm hot and sweaty from the exertion and the pain. I have a catheter in my hand. At this point, the plaster holding it in place slips and the catheter falls out, blood spurting from my hand. The doctors and midwives are too busy with the delivery to stop it. A gauze is chucked at me and I try to hold it in place while continuing to push. Every time I'm distracted by a contraction, the gauze slips again and blood starts squirting from my hand. It's almost comical. There's no point reapplying the plaster – my hand is too sweaty.

The notes say: 'There was a plan to infiltrate the perineum … to perform an episiotomy and expedite the delivery.'

Episiotomy: A cut in the wall of the vagina to create a bigger space for the baby to pass through.

When my rose-tinted spectacles were still intact, I had very much hoped to avoid that word. I didn't want stitches. I didn't want intervention.

But there it is and I do not have a say. I'm told that the doctor will now be performing the procedure to deliver the baby as quickly as possible. I'm not asked, or consulted. It's an emergency. I am told.

◊

So he's coming at me with a pair of scissors. I'm terrified. Lying half-naked on a hospital bed, in the late stages of labour, with my legs suspended in the air and a man coming at me with a knife. I haven't had an epidural. I can still feel everything. Utter terror and panic of the most visceral kind. I feel threatened and under attack. Like a cornered animal.

I panic and shout at him to leave me alone. He, rightly (in retrospect), ignores me. I feel violated. Jamie says this is the only time he's ever heard genuine terror in my voice. I've managed to remain calm and in control until this moment but this is too much. It tips me over the edge and into a state of panic. I don't register who the doctor is, what he looks like. I have a sense of a Frankenstein-like character attacking me. I assume he gave me a local anaesthetic because I feel nothing of the episiotomy, but it's been done.

◊

Thinking about it now, it seems surprising that a doctor could perform an invasive medical procedure on a patient who had just told him forcefully not to do so. It is interesting that he didn't have to gain my permission before doing it. He went against my wishes, as they were at that moment, and he knew it. Yet, he did it anyway. Clearly, it's accepted that in certain circumstances a doctor can make decisions for a patient, and act upon them, without permission. I can see now that there was no time to waste. No time for diplomacy or negotiation. That doctor knew that our baby was in danger and that he had to get her out as soon as possible. Of course, I am glad now that he did that, as stopping to talk me round would have put our daughter at even greater risk.

◊

Almost exactly twenty-four hours after the first contraction, I've become the patient, the victim.

I'm no longer the strong, powerful mother in control of her baby's birth. I'm now completely at the mercy of the situation, the doctors, the midwives, NHS procedures – and of fate.

The wind is taken out of my sails. I'm exhausted and scared and disempowered. So finally, I just give up and lie back in a state of reluctant surrender. I'm now just the object in the middle of a medical drama.

◊

'At 03.56 hours there was a spontaneous vaginal delivery of a live female infant … The emergency bell was activated for a paediatric crash call.'

That's what the medical notes say. The magic of childbirth. The most wonderful moment of a parent's life. All summed up in those words.

I look down. Between my legs I see my baby lying in a pool of blood, amniotic fluid and meconium (a baby's first stool which should be passed after delivery). I feel utterly shellshocked and numb. It is impossible to

18

believe that she has just emerged from my body. What happens next is the real shock, however.

The midwife realises instantly that the baby's in trouble and presses the emergency bell. Paediatricians abandon their duties in A&E and rush to the room. They make it up six floors to Maternity within five minutes. Soon the delivery room is full of people. The baby is whisked off to the resuscitaire, where she's dried and rubbed down before the doctors start to work on her.

Her notes state that she's 'not making respiratory effort'. She isn't breathing. She isn't even trying to breathe. She's floppy, glazed-looking and blue.

At one minute old her Apgar score is three. The NHS uses Apgar scores to define a baby's health and condition at birth. It's a score out of ten, with ten being active, crying, pink, responding to stimulation and with a healthy heart rate. A baby with an Apgar score of between zero and three requires immediate resuscitation. That's where we are.

Jamie

Emma expected that we might struggle to conceive, and this anxiety, borne out of her mother's experience, rubbed off on me. Emma was desperate for a baby and, as a result, we started trying to conceive while we were still relatively young. We didn't want to risk being faced with the double trauma of fertility problems and a ticking biological clock.

Emma was an IVF baby at a time when that was not yet commonplace. She was born only eleven years after Louise Brown, the very first IVF baby.

I know the story well as Emma's dad has always enjoyed opening conversations, and wedding speeches, with: 'Let me tell you about Emma's conception ...' He then goes on to explain to his, usually horrified, audience how she was conceived in a petri dish at the Hallam Medical Centre in London.

Emma was concerned she may have inherited her mother's fertility problems. Her concern rubbed off on me but, as it turned out, she had no problems getting pregnant. Not only was the pregnancy entirely straightforward, but Emma also conceived naturally within a few months of starting to try. We were grateful to have avoided the heartache her parents went through.

Everything having gone so smoothly, and being so low risk, Emma was an obvious candidate for a home birth. It horrifies us now that we could have taken that option. If the baby had been born at home, she would have been dead long before an ambulance could have arrived to whisk her to hospital. Thank goodness we had been clear that we wanted a hospital delivery. Thank goodness she was born in a big, central London hospital where teams of well-equipped medics were constantly present and ready to deal with emergencies.

We are very well aware that had she been born at a small, midwife-led centre, or at a remote cottage hospital, she would probably not have lived. The fact she is here is, in part, down to the fact we lived in London at the time of her birth.

When Emma was pregnant with our second child, a midwife suggested that she might want to have him at our local midwife-led birth centre. As I remember it, Emma looked at her, utterly dumbfounded, laughed and said, 'Have you read my notes?' The idea that we were going to have him anywhere other than in a proper London hospital was laughable.

◊

Emma

I don't see the baby being resuscitated. I can't see her on the other side of the room. All I can see is the huddle of doctors around her.

After twenty-four hours in labour, I'm exhausted. Not a single thought occupies my head. I lie on the bed while the doctors looking after me deliver the placenta and stitch up the episiotomy.

Emotionally, I'm numb and distracted by the injections and stitches I'm being given. I feel them yanking the placenta out. In all the chaos and shock I have somehow forgotten this part of the process. Once the baby is out, I think the whole thing is over. I should be so busy cuddling and admiring my new baby that I shouldn't notice, or care, that the delivery isn't quite over for me.

I assume that the baby is just being cleaned and wrapped up and that she'll then be brought over to me. I've seen on TV babies requiring a little bit of help and am not overly concerned.

I ask whether she is alright and the response I get is: 'We're looking after her.' This doesn't sound like good news. I still don't realise the severity of the situation. My mind isn't clear enough to compute what's happening.

When she's ten minutes old, she is put on a ventilator and is requiring one hundred per cent oxygen to keep her alive. The air we normally breathe is only twenty-one per cent oxygen …

I don't know when I realise just how sick she really is. Maybe it's a gradual realisation. I don't feel a sudden, bombshell moment. Everything happens so fast, it is hard to process it.

After working on her intensively for about half an hour, the doctors bring her over to me momentarily. I get a fleeting glimpse of her and kiss her little forehead before she is whisked off to a critical care cot in the Neonatal Unit on the floor above.

Jamie goes with her and suddenly I find myself alone in the delivery room with the midwife. I feel bad for her because she's been so kind and looked after me so well and I know this is a terrible outcome for her; for her this isn't just a bad day at the office. This will mean investigations. This will mean guilt. This will mean endless questions. She'll never forget this delivery, just as I will never forget it. I feel guilty that we put her in this situation. She doesn't deserve it any more than we do. She deals with it with such dignity and competence. And she continues to look after me so calmly and kindly. She doesn't panic or breakdown; she is a model of professionalism. I have huge respect for her for that. Despite everything that has gone wrong, I don't blame her for a second.

However, I admit to feeling bereft. I'm supposed to be cuddling and feeding my newborn. That's what the books said would happen. Instead, I'm alone. I don't know what's wrong with her. I don't know what's happening to her. I don't even know if she is still alive.

While he is upstairs, Jamie begins writing a diary. A semi-legible account of the day, scrawled on the few free pages of an old notebook. He writes it from her perspective. I asked him later why he did that. He says he doesn't really know, other than he thought he needed to give her a voice. To make her a conscious being. Because conscious beings are permanent.

He writes:

> 'My Daddy (who loves me more than anything in the world) is there to see me when I come out.
> 'I am all squished and after a few minutes am trying very hard to breathe but I can only manage a little gurgle.
> 'Daddy says this is a very sad moment for him because he can see I'm trying so hard but that I'm struggling. He says that he knows at that moment he will love me forever and always look after me.
> 'Even though I'm trying very hard, the kind midwives and doctors have to look after me. The room is full of very important people. Obviously,

23

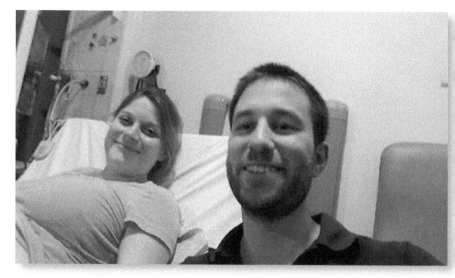

Jamie and Emma at the Royal Free Hospital during the labour

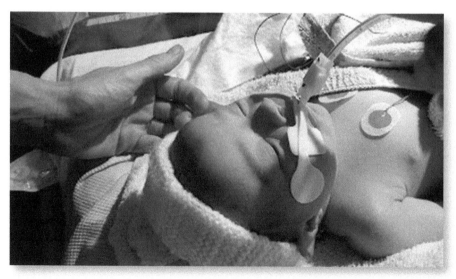

The first photo taken of Sophie when she was just minutes old. It was taken in the delivery room by Jamie

they mostly come to see just how cute I am. But they also know I need help and they take me upstairs for special treatment.

'My daddy comes upstairs with me to help look after me. On the way up we get to look into each other's eyes, and I recognise him straight away because he has so much love in his eyes for me.

'Daddy tells me that it is the best moment of his life, looking into my eyes. He says I'm his little soldier because I am fighting so hard to live.'

Below this, Jamie draws a circle around a smudge on the page. Next to it, it says:

'One of Daddy's tears because he's sad to see me so unwell.'

Chapter Three

*I*n the Neonatal Unit the baby is diagnosed with meconium aspiration syndrome, sepsis, persistent pulmonary hypertension of the neonate and HIE Grade Two.

The doctors think she developed an infection during the labour and that it progressed so rapidly that she had sepsis by the time she was delivered. I tested positive for group B strep (a usually harmless bacteria present in almost half of the population which can, occasionally, be passed to babies during birth) but she didn't. It's possible she has group B strep but, if so, it doesn't behave typically in her. It is never established exactly what infection she has or how she acquired it. The important thing is that she has an infection and it's bad.

Unbeknown to anyone, she was also being starved of oxygen for hours during the labour for reasons that remain unexplained. Possibly the placenta was failing. No one knows. As a result, she has HIE – hypoxic-ischaemic encephalopathy. In layman's terms, brain damage caused by oxygen deprivation. There are four grades of HIE, one being the least severe and four the most severe. Our baby has grade two HIE.

Due to the oxygen deprivation and the infection, she became distressed during the labour. The distress caused her to pass meconium before she was delivered. The infection also meant she started gulping and trying to take her first breath before she was born. So, she aspirated a lot of meconium and developed exceptionally severe meconium aspiration syndrome. Meconium has the consistency of tar, so her lungs are full of this awful, sticky substance which strips the lining of the lungs and makes it impossible for her to breathe.

She was unable to take a breath when she was delivered so she also developed persistent pulmonary hypertension.

When a baby is in the womb, they don't need to use their lungs because they get all the oxygen they need through the umbilical cord. The blood vessels that take blood from the heart to the lungs are closed. When a baby takes their first breath, these blood vessels open meaning oxygenated blood can be taken from the lungs to the heart. As our baby didn't take a first breath, this didn't happen, and the blood vessels remained closed. This is persistent pulmonary hypertension.[1] It isn't glamorous or well known, but it is very dangerous.

She is less than an hour old and already diagnosed with four separate conditions, each of which is life-threatening.

Once she is sedated and ventilated, she is as stable as they can make her. Her life is no longer in imminent danger. So the doctors turn their attention to her brain. Her poor, oxygen-starved brain. Should she survive, protecting her brain is vital for her long-term prognosis. Therefore, they begin cooling her whole body – reducing her body temperature to thirty-three degrees – in a bid to protect her brain from further damage. They achieve this by lying her on pads of cold water.

Technically, this process is known as induced therapeutic hypothermia, or active cooling. It's the equivalent for the brain of putting an ice pack on a sprained ankle to prevent swelling. This is particularly crucial in the case of brain injury because the brain is in such an enclosed space. If it swells too much it is constricted by the skull, which increases the pressure inside the skull and can be fatal.

Cooling is a relatively new treatment option for babies who have been deprived of oxygen and so research into it is ongoing. However, it is also thought to reduce the number of brain cells that die following oxygen deprivation. It aims to reduce the death rate from HIE and, also, to reduce the risk of lifelong disability.[2]

When they have done all they can for her, the doctors have to decide how to proceed. She can't stay at our local hospital, The Royal Free. She needs specialist care. The consultant speaks to the local neonatal intensive care units (NICUs) – at Great Ormond Street Hospital (GOSH) and University College London Hospital (UCLH) – to discuss the best course of action. Initially, they fear she will have to be placed on heart-lung bypass (ECMO). In that case, cooling could not continue, but stopping it would affect her long-term prognosis, should she survive.

In the end, the NICU at UCLH agrees to attempt to sustain her on a ventilator so she can continue the cooling. The absolute priority is keeping her alive, but the doctors are also mindful of achieving the best long-term prognosis.

All that is left for The Royal Free to do is to organise her transfer to the NICU at UCLH. This involves booking a London Neonatal Transfer Service (NTS) ambulance. There are only three available and they are busy.

Chapter Four

There are hours between the delivery and the baby leaving in the ambulance. Maybe five? I don't know for sure. Time comes to me as a series of snapshots. Disconnected, but significant, moments between which everything is a blur.

Once the baby has been moved upstairs, and the doctors have finished stitching me up, I look around the empty delivery room and wonder what to do next. In happier circumstances I would be engrossed in trying to master the art of breastfeeding a newborn. As it is, I have no role. No job. I can't be a mother to my baby; I don't even know where exactly she is.

I should be sending excited messages to everyone with pictures of her. In reality, it doesn't occur to me to contact anyone. What would I say to them? I don't have any pictures to share, I don't know how she is, I don't know what's wrong with her …

If she were with me, I might consider having a nap once she'd gone to sleep. After all, I've been awake for more than twenty-four hours. But it isn't the time for that. I'm not sleepy. I can't relax after the rigours of the birth because I don't know what's happening. I'm waiting.

I'm waiting to be told if my baby is alive. If she is going to live. What is wrong with her.

During this void, while the doctors upstairs are battling to stabilise her, the midwife suggests I have a shower. It is a good point. I'm half-naked and covered in sweat and blood.

Hospital showers are horrible. Clinical and unfriendly and unwelcoming. Together with that, there's a sense that they're probably not very clean. That a lot of other blood- and sweat-soaked people have used them before you. That they are there to clean dirty bodies, covered in unsavoury bodily fluids, rather than to be luxuriated in. However, there's no option. I have to have a shower and put clean clothes on. I can't remain in the state I'm in. Maybe I'll feel more human after a shower.

The lovely midwife helps me hobble to the bathroom. She helps me shower my filthy, exhausted, newly stitched and bleeding body. I watch the blood dripping onto the shower floor, mixing with the water and swirling down the plughole.

Perhaps because of shock, I'm completely calm and collected and rational and sensible. I don't scream or cry or get hysterical. Panicked thoughts don't crash through my mind. My brain needs a chance to process everything that's happened before it can involve itself emotionally. I just get on with showering a body that, hours earlier, had been fit and healthy and strong and nourishing a full-term baby. I am shocked by the way it has changed so fast. At the toll the birth has taken. I'm almost afraid of it, as if I don't know who, or quite what, it is anymore.

Washing my hair makes me feel better. I feel clean again. I'm conscious that it's necessary. It seems an odd moment, and setting, in which to be washing and conditioning, but I have to. My hair is filthy.

Clean and wet, I stagger gingerly out of the bathroom, afraid of tearing stitches and of more pain and more blood. I put on clean pyjamas and a dressing gown and eat a slice of NHS toast and jam.

I'm sitting on the bed staring absentmindedly out of the window when Jamie returns. He is torn. Our baby is fighting for her life in the neonatal unit. His wife, who has just given birth, is alone in the delivery room. His position is impossible. He's needed in two places at the same time. In two brutal places.

He is, however, calm and loving and supportive. He's doing his best to support both of us. I'm glad when he's with me. But I am also content with him not being by my side if that means he's with our baby. He's not just her father but her advocate. I trust him entirely to love her and to look after her in any way he can. Knowing he is with her means I don't need to feel guilty that I can't yet be by her side.

The Maternity Department walls are plastered with posters extolling the virtues of breastfeeding and skin-to-skin contact for newborns. Posters designed to make the parents who can't offer their baby those things feel guilty.

Healthy mothers with healthy babies offer those things anyway. It's natural, instinctive. They don't need to be told. They don't need posters to remind them. I look at the posters and feel guilty. But it isn't my fault. My baby needs breastfeeding and she needs skin-to-skin and she needs the comfort and reassurance of being held by her mother, but she needs life-saving medical care even more than she needs those things and the two are mutually exclusive.

Jamie and I sit in silence, completely bewildered and confused. Jamie back on the chair by the window. Me on the newly cleaned bed. In just the same positions as earlier in the night. Except everything has changed. Then, we had thought we were about to welcome a healthy baby. Now, the baby is gone. She isn't with me for the first time since the moment of her conception. We don't know what's happening to her. We don't know if we'll ever take her home. If we do, we don't know what life will look like for her.

I picture the lovingly prepared Moses basket sitting beside our bed at home. Empty. Empty but for the pink comforter we had put in it. How long will it remain empty for? Perhaps it will always be empty?

I turn to Jamie and say: 'I don't feel very hopeful about her.'

He just nods.

I've given up now and I feel guilty about that. But I've never seen her. I've had only a fleeting glance. I don't know how beautiful she is. I don't know how strong and robust

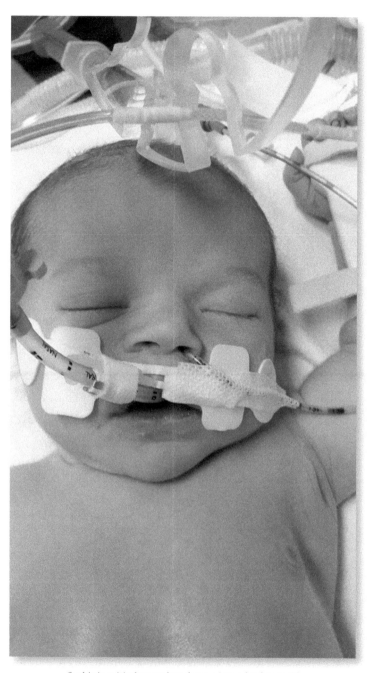

Sophie in critical care when she was just a few hours old

she looks. I don't have an image to cling on to. I don't know who it is I am willing to survive. I don't know her.

Unlike me, Jamie has seen her properly. Jamie witnessed the birth in HD.

I'm too dazed by pain, hormones, gas and air to be fully conscious of what's been happening. I was wrapped up in what was happening inside my body, and with trying to cope with the labour and delivery. I wasn't watching the facial expressions of the medics.

But Jamie was.

I wasn't listening to their every worried word.

Jamie was. He knew things were bad before I did and he witnessed the whole disaster play out in horrifying detail. He remembers it clearly and he looks haunted.

◊

I don't remember Sophie's delivery nearly as clearly as Jamie does because of the hormones and medication I was on. So, I've asked Jamie to give a full account of it.

Jamie

Sophie sneaks into the sitting-room-converted-to-office for the Covid-19 lockdown of 2020. I can hear her padding up to me and can sense the mischievous smile on her face.

I pretend not to hear. Never spoil a good game.

She says 'boo' and presents her most recent collection of drawings. I pull her onto my lap – all four years of her gorgeous self.

Gosh, she is getting big! I hold her close and give her a cuddle.

She giggles and squirms. 'Daddy, your cold nose is tickling me'.

She's my talisman to shield me from the unpleasantness of going back to the raw emotions of her birth.

Deep breath.

I dread going back to those emotions. Those still frames and moving pictures stuck in my mind, resistant to time. The choking sounds. The fear and panic. The disconnected feeling of mind, body and reality. Emma's calm, trusting eyes, despite everything. Sophie's beautiful eyes looking into mine for the first time.

Not yet.

Start typing.

◊

Emma's recollection of the birth is very different to mine. She remembers the physical sensations she was experiencing but her memory of it is also hazy. I recollect it as an observer with a clear head. I want to describe what it was like for me.

We had our own room. It looked just like your average hospital room. There was a large black window reflecting our images. The rest becomes hazy.

Time doesn't operate normally in such circumstances. For a start it was late. There was that dream-like disorientation one can get after landing in a foreign airport in the dark. I remember trying to say silly things, or make naughty comments, about waders, plungers and goggles to cheer Emma up. I'm never sure whether she actually finds my jokes funny but I can't resist telling them. If nothing else, I think she enjoys rolling her eyes at me and playing the disapproving wife.

Our midwife had dark hair, quite young, perhaps slightly inexperienced, but friendly and reassuring.

I remember the contractions getting fiercer. As they grew in power the pain began to overwhelm Emma. Her eyes rolled in panic. Her voice became desperate. Her breathing erratic. I found my role – to hold her head close to me and look her in the eyes during a contraction. To talk calmly, to reassure her just to breathe and it would pass. She took gas and air for pain relief. She calmed down and found her own rhythm. She was doing a fantastic job. I was so proud of her. It was scary to see the woman I love in pain like that.

I think fathers are poorly prepared. Society has removed gore and violence too effectively. The birthing books and NCT groups give more emphasis to empowerment and involvement. They tend to gloss over the fact that childbirth is painful, gory and potentially dangerous. It's watching your most loved friend be tortured by their own body at a time when they are most vulnerable, while having no real control, role or emotional preparation for the experience. I think society has created a role for the twenty-first-century father which is quite simply unbalanced. It romanticises the positives and does nothing to prepare you or to offer follow-up advice. You get a horror movie in 4K definition with your partner as the protagonist.

I remember the midwife hooking Emma up to the mobile foetus ECG machine to monitor our baby's heart rate. I remember the printer in the corner of the room gently oozing a steady stream of graphs. I remember quizzing the midwife about it and asking what she was looking for. Everything seemed normal. Heart rate dropped during contractions, then recovered. There are certain warning signs around this pattern that they look for – something to do with the speed and regularity with which the heart rate recovers. For our night shift all seemed well. Emma was dilating further. Six centimetres. Eight centimetres. The senior midwife came in to check every now and then. She was quite brusque and grumpy. Just another shift. More fretting first-timers nagging her. Nothing to see here. Emma would wander around the room and try different positions to ride out the contractions – ECG cables tagging behind her like a dog on a lead.

I remember it getting very late. Emma had been told earlier on that they would expect her to take six to eight hours to dilate fully. She was shocked. The reality was that between the rhythms of the contractions, the hormones coursing through her body, and the gas and air, time flowed differently for her. She asked what the time was and when I said 1am her jaw dropped. She thought twenty minutes had passed.

I remember eating a Mars bar. I looked out of the window northward. The sky was dark. Most of the lights were off, and I could make out the greater darkness of Hampstead Heath. It was a friendly scene, but one from which I felt strangely removed.

We were nearing the delivery. The senior midwife was coming in to check the heart rate more often. The consultant popped in to see how things were going. At some point Emma got to ten centimetres. The midwife could feel the head. We were in business. Now it was time to start pushing through the contractions. I was excited. We were getting there, and my darling wife was doing it all herself. It was textbook, and we would soon reach that magical moment when the baby pops out, you hear a cry, and they're placed with a towel over them on the mother's chest. When all the darkness, uncertainty, and unfathomableness of the universe is swept aside. A moment of sudden recognition of what it is to bring life into the world. Emma's deepest yearnings fulfilled, and in her deepest joy I would be complete.

Progress should have been swift. We all took turns to help encourage Emma to push. The midwife was great. The senior one came in to add her advice and check the monitor. We weren't to know of the crisis unfolding right before us in our little girl. Some of the clues were there to see already.

I don't remember how or when it happened, but like an old weathervane suddenly creaking to signal an ominous change in wind direction the mood started to darken. To become more nervous. To become a bit more urgent. I can't remember if it was said, and whether it was the senior midwife or consultant, but the sense was 'it's time to get this baby out'. Nature could no longer be relied on. Was this shift rapid or slow? I can't remember. Perhaps the medical notes would provide a more objective account of the events.

What I do know is that I started to feel afraid. Not the abstract something-might-happen anxiety. That sinking feeling in the gut. Something is wrong. Something bad is unfolding here.

I pause in my writing. Dry sobs rack through me even four years later because of what was to come.

The midwives were now encouraging Emma to push. That was the strategy to get the baby moving. The consultant came in more frequently. The ECG was looked at more often. I leaned in closer to Emma – the instinct to protect drawing me to her side. My focus became to look after her and to try to shield her from what I could see unfolding before me. I tried to get answers when she couldn't hear. What were they worried about? Emma was thankfully completely engrossed in the birth – the long process of labour and the mind state it seems to produce protecting her from the hard realities of what was happening to her body and within that room.

The moment of crisis was near. Despite Emma's best efforts, the baby wasn't moving forward. She appeared to be stuck. I was desperately sad because Emma was just so perfect. She was doing all this so stoically and lovingly. She never complained. She did exactly what she should have done. She should have had her perfect victory because she deserved it, but nature and circumstance had whipped all that away from her.

Now the consultant was in the room the whole time, the three medical staff outnumbering us. The consultant, I think, was in his thirties. He sounded Greek, had black hair and dark-rimmed glasses. Whatever was concerning him finally resolved in his mind, and he decided to perform an emergency episiotomy. Emma was lain on the bed in that way you see in movies, lying on her back, legs open and bent. He got the scalpel. Emma screamed in terror. 'No! Get off me. Get off me.' I couldn't look. I was standing at the top of the bed by my darling wife's left ear as she was cut. I held my head close to her. I whispered what I could to calm her. I hope I told her I loved her.

What happened next was the most powerful series of images and moments that I've ever experienced. The consultant was now able to wrench the baby out. It all happened so quickly. Like the violent resolution to a Tarantino film. It was all the more potent because the moment of delivery and glory was actually a nightmare.

Out came our daughter. I knew something was wrong though I was not yet able to process it. It really was like watching a film. A surreal, grotesque, out-of-body experience.

Blood. Lots. On the white sheets. My wife's guts, or parts of them. Lots of thick, brown, churned up, frothy fluid. Like the rain-filled grooves made by a tractor tyre in a muddy field. My daughter there in the middle of this mess. A baby, but she looked swollen and blotchy. A blueish hue. Were her eyes open?

I hope to God this memory is a creative embellishment of the mind.

She looked like she was being throttled by invisible blood-drenched hands. Eyes straining open. I waited for that piercing cry. That shriek that life is beginning as air fills the lungs. Instead, there was choking. Gurgling. Like a small animal trapped in a drain.

This wasn't right. I was caught between a mix of shock and curiosity. I knew but couldn't know. There but a million miles away. This was as real as it gets and yet it felt like a figment of my imagination. This couldn't be happening. I felt like a helpless avatar watching. Unable to move. Just to watch. I remember feeling: 'This is interesting. This is like when things go wrong. Let's see what happens'.

Fortunately, the medical staff were not in this daze. The senior midwife took the baby and started the initial steps of trying to get her to breathe. Rubbing the back, the swinging motion. Thumping the chest. I must have asked if she was okay and what was wrong? I don't remember the response. The answer was in their panicked tone of voice, the urgency of their movements. Many things must have been happening all at once but I could only see this little baby failing to live. The truth was screaming at us. The noise absolutely silent.

I don't remember anything dramatic being shouted, but the consultant said something, the senior midwife ran to the wall. Within seconds the room was full of people. I was still standing next to Emma where I'd been before. An eternity ago. Is it called a code blue? I don't know. It feels as if it has nothing to do with me. And yet, of course, it absolutely does.

The medics took our daughter to the incubator in the corner. A consultant in a mask, googles and with a light on his head, started to lean over and work on her. A cruel, bright, white light was turned on. It was cruel because it was so sharp, and because it laid bare the reality of the situation. Still the choking gurgling. The scene in that corner seemed like a cheap pub carvery – with a large lump of undercooked meat under the bright glare of the warming lamp, with some nightmarish chef prodding and carving the joint. Juices flowing. This was our magical moment, upended.

The consultant was using an instrument that looked a bit like a dentist's suction pipe. He was working quickly and methodically to flush out the thick, brown, visceral fluid that had saturated her face, nose, mouth, throat and lungs. Brown fluid gushed everywhere. The sounds were even worse than what I could see. Sucking, gurgling, spraying, gurgling, choking. Death was waiting in that room and there was no dignity or mercy. The initial shock must have passed because I became aware of what I was watching, and I was aware my wife was lying next to me in a bed covered in her own blood and guts. A consultant was getting ready to stitch her up. I couldn't bear to see what was happening to my daughter and I'd never felt so helpless. I think at that moment I knew quite clearly that she was dying on the little table next to us. It was only a matter of time.

One clear thought came to mind. *Look after Emma*. Even in that moment of crisis and loss I felt I must protect my wife. I have always felt a need to protect her. She was so young when we started going out, having just left school. I was in the year above her at university, she was new to that environment and to life outside her sheltered girls' school. I was a year older and had a little more life experience. I felt a responsibility to look after her then, and now. Always.

Emma had done everything right. From the start of the pregnancy to the end she had done everything with love and everything to give our baby the best start. She had gone into labour bravely and had shown the best forms of courage and love that a mother could show. I felt bitterly sad and angry that she might forever blame herself for what we had lost when she had done everything right. Some perpetual purgatory of survivor's guilt.

Emma was perfectly calm. Her face poised. So beautiful. People don't need to be strong all the time to have unconquerable strength in them. In a quiet, slightly sad, but caring and loving voice, she turned to me from her bed to ask: 'What's happening. How is she?'

I don't know what I said. I think it was that the doctors were looking after her. She was struggling to breathe. I told her I loved her. That she had done everything right. That I was so proud of her.

Emma was so dignified. She was so calm. I think we embraced. One of those embraces where warmth and love seem to cement you together. Where words seem insignificant and unnecessary.

What happened next? How long did this go on for? I don't really know.

The consultant kept working on our child. I don't know who he was – I should know his name. There's no doubt that his actions saved her life. There's no way she was going to last for five minutes without the team desperately trying to open up her airways and get oxygen into her blue, sluggish body.

Time passed.

I think they put an oxygen mask on her. She started to look a little pinker. The noises coming from her became a little bit less desperate.

At the same time, Emma was being stitched up. The room was still full of doctors and nurses. We found out later that basically every paediatrician and A&E doctor in the hospital had been scrambled to help. Even the on-call consultants at home were urgently rushed to the hospital to assist. At the time, our baby must have been the sickest person in north west London.

I kept holding Emma's hand, and tried to find the right words to reassure her. It was the only thing I could think to do.

The initial crisis had passed, but clearly we weren't out of the woods yet. They were transferring our baby to an incubatory trolley with oxygen mask on because she needed to be in their critical care unit.

Emma was in no position to move anywhere, but I could go with them. I must have squeezed Emma's hand and kissed her goodbye. It was all a bit of a daze. Not the procession of triumph we were hoping for. We went in the medical-staff-only lifts.

During this transition I have one crystal-clear recollection. The only beautiful moment in all this mess.

Our baby was lying on her tummy, with her head facing to the right. Her eyes were open. I moved around the trolley as they waited for the lift so I could see her. I looked into her eyes for the first time. They were so beautiful. A little bit bleary and red, but gorgeous. They looked chestnut-brown at the time. We had a moment where our eyes connected. I am certain she was aware and that she saw me. I think in that moment I knew her. In that moment I fell irrevocably in love with her. She was so close to death that her life was somehow even more potent. I swear I could see her little soul in her eyes.

I think it is at this point that my memory starts to fail me. The shock and vividness of the situation was replaced by a duller series of events. They sedated her and spent some time trying to stabilise her. I was sent down to Emma as there wasn't space by the bed, and I think the situation was sufficiently urgent that they needed to be on their own to work.

Chapter Five

Emma

The delivery room door opens. In walks a column of doctors. A senior consultant flanked by junior doctors and nurses. Their faces paint a grim picture. They look utterly downcast and solemn. None of this bodes well.

I honestly believe they are going to tell us she has died. I think I have accepted the fact, for this moment at least.

◊

Jamie

I went to Emma. Tiredness and shock set in. Numbness. Loss.

After Emma was stitched up we were moved to a postnatal recovery room with no baby to recover with. The room was dark.

5am.

6am.

We were so close. Physically and emotionally. Then, the darkest moment of my life. Four doctors came quietly into the room. It was only partially lit by the early dawn outside. The moment we had been preparing for had come. We were now going to be told that she had died. Their body language. The context. They might as well just nod and leave.

◊

Emma

Instead, the consultant, who has wild, frizzy, ginger hair, a strong German accent and is wearing green checked leggings, gives us an update. I never normally notice what anyone is wearing. Is her appearance just particularly notable? Maybe I imagined it. I don't know.

She explains what is wrong with the baby. Tells us that they have sucked as much of the meconium from her lungs as they can and that they've put her on a ventilator. She says that she is in discussions with two major NICUs; then she reassures us that they're doing their best for our baby and that she will let us know as soon as they have decided on a concrete course of action. She tells us that she is sorry to say she 'can't predict a good outcome'.

Then they leave. They go back to her. They go back to trying to save her life. That handful of people are her only chance of a future. They're our only chance of keeping our baby. Her life is in their hands. They have been fighting so hard to keep her alive that, for more than an hour, they haven't even had a chance to tell me, her mother, what is happening.

I'm ashamed to say that I don't even know their names. I don't know who it is that steps up in the middle of the night to help us when we need them most. But they do, those amazing people are there and doing everything they possibly can for her, despite believing that it's hopeless.

It's four in the morning. They were probably expecting a quiet night in paediatric A&E. Maybe a few babies with croup, maybe the odd high fever, a child with a cut lip …

And then, out of the blue, their emergency buzzer sounds. They fly up six floors to the Maternity Department and find themselves flung, without warning, into a desperate life-or-death struggle. Into a situation where a baby's life is entirely in their hands. Into the rawest, most desperate situation. They have to tell new parents that their baby is probably going to die. They have to fight to save her, and to deliver earth-shattering news at the same time. Then, I assume, they wash their hands, have breakfast and go to bed, only to be ready to do it all again the following night, if needed.

◊

Through some bizarre coincidence, about six months later, Jamie's sister met one of the junior doctors who helped resuscitate our baby. Natalie was chatting to a fellow tourist when she was on holiday in Israel and he mentioned that he was a paediatrician at the Royal Free

Hospital. Natalie explained that her niece had been born there a few months previously and that she'd been very unwell. They soon established that this man was one of the doctors who had looked after her. He told Natalie that she was one of the sickest babies he had ever seen. He had looked after her at the most critical moment of her illness, but he had no idea what had happened to her after she had left the Royal Free at a few hours old. He didn't know whether his actions had been enough to save her life. Natalie showed him some pictures and videos of our baby as she was then – six months old. He cried.

◊

Once again, Jamie and I are alone with our thoughts. Helpless. With no role. We can only wait while the doctors work on her and help her tiny, vulnerable, newborn body to fight this battle.

Chapter Six

A receptionist walks into the room. At least, I assume she's a receptionist. Maybe she's a midwife? She tells me my mother has called, worried about me. Oh, God! Yes! Mum. We had been texting her earlier in the night. We had told her I was in labour and that I'd been admitted to the Labour Ward. I think Jamie had even told her the birth was imminent. She must be expecting a joyful update. Her first grandchild. A granddaughter born to her only daughter. Instead, we have gone completely silent. She must be beside herself with worry. She must have spent the night lying in bed awake waiting for updates and wondering how we were getting on. Whether everything was okay.

In the chaos and the shock of the aftermath of the birth, I have completely forgotten to update her. I'm not putting off calling her or wondering what to say. I just don't think to call her.

The receptionist, if she is a receptionist, has told Mum that she can't tell her anything because of patient confidentiality. But she assured Mum that she would ask me to contact her. I now know that she is worried and that I need to call her. So, without being entirely rational, that's what I do. However, it isn't the best moment. After you've had a baby, the midwife is very keen to see that you are still able to go for a wee. And that's what I am doing – I am trying to prove that I can still pass urine.

Even worse, they make you wee into a cardboard pot which they put inside the loo so you can present the evidence that your bladder still works. So, when I call her, I am sitting on the loo, over a cardboard pot full of wee and blood.

I think this is the single most vulnerable moment of my life. I have just given birth for the first time. I am naked and bleeding. And I am calling my mother to tell her that her first grandchild is in critical care. Why I don't wait five minutes before calling her, I have no idea.

'Mum, it's me. The baby is out. Don't worry about me – I'm fine – but she's not doing very well. She couldn't breathe. They are looking after her upstairs.'

That's what I tell her. I then go on to explain that they are still trying to decide where to transfer her and that I will let her know as soon as I do. Then we discuss logistics. We agree she will come up and meet me in the Maternity Department.

She doesn't ask me many questions and she is right not to. I don't know the answers. We're both just being practical and working out what to do next with the limited information we have. We are aware that, when the baby is transferred, Jamie will go with her. I probably won't be able to. So, Mum will come and keep me company on the Postnatal Ward.

I am very grateful to Mum for coming to be with me. I feel intensely vulnerable and need help showering, cleaning my episiotomy stitches and packing my things. Who better than my own mum? I can't look after my daughter, but she can look after hers. There is no one else, other than Jamie, I would feel comfortable with seeing me naked and helping me with those very personal tasks. Mum was in a unique position to help.

Chapter Seven

*A*t some point around breakfast time – maybe about two hours after the birth, maybe slightly longer – someone asks me if I would like to go and see the baby. Clearly, she is deemed stable enough and I fit enough. I haven't asked to see her. I'm just waiting to be told what to do. I'm now a passenger on this journey. I don't have the energy to express my own opinions, or even to have any. I'm too exhausted, physically and emotionally, after the labour. I'm happy to be guided by the staff. It's easier.

In my dressing gown and slippers, I'm wheeled out of Maternity. I think that I could perfectly well walk. I feel self-conscious being stuck in a wheelchair. The midwife takes me up in the lift, and into Paediatrics.

At the end of a corridor of brightly painted walls, through lots of doors, is the Neonatal Unit. I'm wheeled up to the critical care cot where my baby is lying, while a sweet-faced nurse and a couple of doctors potter around attending to her. The initial frenzied work of stabilising her is over and the room is calm.

She has a ventilator stuck down her throat, held in place by a big, white plaster across her face. She has splints and cuffs and plasters and wires attached to both arms and hands; she has multicoloured wires coming out of her heavily-bandaged umbilical cord stump. She's naked except for a nappy. There are syringes of fluid beside her. There is one big spot of her blood on the otherwise pristine white sheet she is lying on.

I look at the nurse and breathe: 'Wow! She's beautiful.'

The nurse replies: 'Yes. She really is.'

She says it as though she means it and I'm touched.

She's perfect. A perfectly formed, plump, eight-pound baby. She looks so strong and robust and healthy. She looks like she would be in perfect health if you pulled all the wires and tubes out. She doesn't look as if she needs them. She shouldn't need them. If she had been delivered by caesarean section a few days earlier, she'd probably be free of them. Yet, without them she would die almost instantly.

She's sedated. Her beautiful almond-shaped eyes, with their enviable, long, dark eyelashes, are closed. She has a full head of dark hair, an adorable button nose and soft, pink cheeks. She's just perfect. She is all I could ever have dreamt of and I desperately want to be able to keep her. I want to see her beautiful little face without the tubes and plasters. I want to hold her and to cuddle her and to look after her, but I can't. I wipe away the tears that are rolling down my face with the corner of my dressing gown. I don't have a tissue.

All sense of hopelessness disappears once I've seen her. She's real to me now. A real person, a real baby. My baby.

She looks so pink and healthy and strong. She can't die. Surely, she can't? People who look so well don't just die. Do they?

The nurse asks us whether we have a name for her. Her notes refer to her as Baby Innes as does the label on her incubator. She needs a name. She needs an identity. Names give permanence. We can't let her die without a name. Somehow, the lack of a name makes her feel transient.

We have a shortlist, but we haven't decided. We thought we would wait and see what she was like before making our decision. Mull it over while cuddling and admiring her. Now there's an urgency. She needs a name before any more notes refer to her as 'Baby Innes'. We're horrified by the idea of her dying without a name.

The nurse suggests that she looks like an Olivia. I agree. She does look like an Olivia. That isn't right, though. Then her initials would be Oi! That wouldn't do. We consider Charlotte but it doesn't really go with our surname. I suggest Sophie. Yes. That feels right. It is pretty and sweet, just like she is. We tell the doctors authoritatively that she is now called Sophie. No more 'Baby Innes'. She has a name.

Sophie.

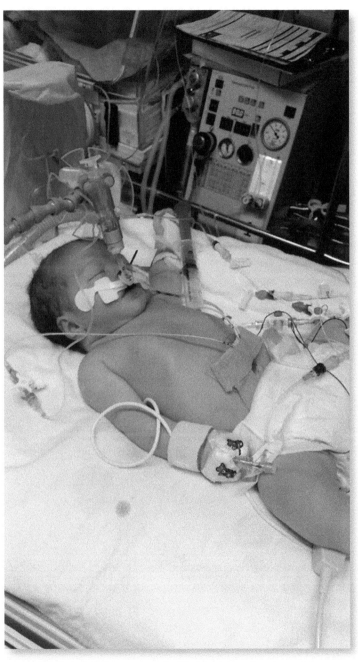

*The first photo Emma ever took of Sophie – taken when she went to
see her in critical care. It was the first time she saw her properly*

Chapter Eight

While I'm with her, the transfer ambulance arrives. It's staffed by a paramedic, a neonatal consultant and a neonatal intensive care nurse and it contains more sophisticated equipment than the hospital does. The team enter the room with a cheery air. They're warm and friendly and reassuring.

The hospital begins to hand Sophie's care over to the transfer team who carry out a further suction of her lungs and give her some physio to help shift the fluid in them. This improves her oxygenation. They also transfer her onto their ventilator and increase the degree of cooling she's receiving.

Jamie's diary, in Sophie's voice

'I am so lovely and special, they arranged for an amazing, specialist ambulance to collect me.

'The midwife and doctors who looked after me in the delivery room came to say goodbye to me.

'Daddy is very excited because the ambulance put its lights and sirens on in order to get me to the neonatal intensive care unit as quickly as possible.'

◊

I sit in my wheelchair and watch as my new, critically ill, baby is wheeled out of the room in a covered incubator, followed by my husband. They leave without me. I can't go with them because I'm still a patient of the Maternity Department. I have to wait to be discharged; have to remember that I, too, am a patient; have to trust other people to look after her when she needs it most.

The nurse reassures me that they will cover her incubator with a blanket to protect her privacy as she is wheeled through the hospital to the ambulance. I'm surprised by this comment. It's touching that they are thinking not only of her immediate medical needs, but also of her dignity. It just hasn't occurred to me as an issue. It is a nice touch. It would seem wrong for strangers to be staring at her as she lies fighting for her life in an incubator wearing nothing but a nappy.

◊

To this day, I get goosebumps when I see an ambulance screeching through London on blue lights. I can no longer look at ambulances dispassionately. I can't help but wonder about the human story behind the sirens. I know what it's like to be on the wrong side of an ambulance. I know that hundreds of Londoners must have witnessed the NTS ambulance fly through Camden to UCLH with Sophie inside. Now I understand that these sirens mean another family is facing a life-or-death emergency, just as we did.

◊

Once they have left, the midwife kindly takes me back downstairs to wait for Mum and then to be discharged so that I can join my baby in the NICU at UCLH.

She takes me back to Maternity but not, this time, to the delivery room. They need the delivery room for someone else. She takes me to the Postnatal Ward. To a private bereavement room. A room where they put women who have just given birth but who do not have a baby. Once again, I am alone. Alone in a bereavement room. But I am not bereaved yet, am I? There is still hope.

I sit on the bed, waiting for Mum and staring at my phone in case Jamie sends me an update. I'm entirely dependent upon him to keep my informed as to what's happening to Sophie. I just have to trust that he'll relay any important news. I have to keep believing that if she's died, he would have told me. I have to keep reassuring myself that, to use the old cliché, no news is probably good news. That, as no one has told me otherwise, she must still be fighting.

◊

I didn't go in the transfer ambulance so I asked Jamie to describe this part of the story.

Jamie

'At night our fear is strong, but in the morning, in the light, we find our courage again.' Ziauddin Yousafzai.[3]

60

I feel able to write these words not only because Emma has instructed me to, but also because, at this point in the story, there was the beginning of hope, although not the end of fear. The plummet down the abyss was over. Maybe now we could look up and see the still sky above. Good stories always have heroes, so I'll start with the first of mine: the London NTS team who attended to Sophie early on the morning of her birth. Three people I'd never met before and have never seen again. They represented the best of London, the best of the NHS, and the best of what it means to show humanity to those who need it.

They were the best of London because of their diverse backgrounds and resilient characters. The talented, Germanic calm of the European doctor and the classic Blitz-spirit East Londoner paramedic/driver, Mick, with his cheery patter and absolute dependency. They must have had ten years of medical training between them to get to where they were, and many more years of on-the-job experience. Jerome the doctor, whose country of origin was not obvious, but he was probably continental European. He didn't look like your typical doctor. Tall, grey-black hair, long and in dreadlocks. Probably good at an arm wrestle. The specialist neonatal nurse, Zak.

The incubator they hooked Sophie up to was, quite literally, a miniaturised ICU. It resembled something that might emerge from a space capsule. All of it to keep our little daughter, who we had just met, alive.

So many people to make it possible. So much money from society collectively to pay for it.

They resembled the best of humanity because not only did they give our baby their talented care, but they also treated us with courtesy, respect, honesty and optimism. Surely this small team, which could fit into one ambulance, is what society, social media and our collective institutions should be holding up as the epitome of what we should all strive to be and value?

These were the cavalry, our knights in shining armour. We know from acquaintances that our 'birthing experience' was quite an unusual and extreme event for the staff on the Royal Free's Maternity Ward. We heard that for a member of the emergency team at the crash call, it was the worst experience he had had in all his years of service.

The hospital team had managed to keep her alive, but they were right at the edge of their expertise, experience, and equipment. We owe them a lot for taking on such an extreme and unexpected emergency, and for keeping her alive. But it very much felt like damage limitation, while this was right up the NTS team's street.

The NTS were the A Team. They had done this all before. They knew it was bad, but they had seen worse. They knew that babies are both vulnerable and remarkably resilient, and that while there's moving red blood in those arteries then there's hope.

By breakfast time, they had managed to further stabilise her, and she had started to almost resemble a pink, breathing baby again, despite the multitude of tubes, wires and tapes surrounding her. They radiated a particular kind of calm and positivity to which I cannot remotely do justice. How they managed it, I still have no idea.

All I can say is that I have never taken greater comfort in a terrible situation than when I walked into the Neonatal Unit and they were there. What was the feeling? There was now hope. The grieving process we had both started could wait. We had braced ourselves several times for the dreaded softly spoken words. Not Yet. Our child was still to be fought for.

I am writing this without the aid of my diary or the medical notes. Tangible medical things were happening. But this is about feelings, and the shift from abject loss and horror to the beginning of hope was one of the defining emotional experiences of my life.

The details were vague because the experience was so removed from reality. We were travelling through a disembodied dreamworld. Only the feelings really stand out clearly. I remember the doctors discussing her condition, Jerome on the phone in his calm way, organising where she should be transferred to. Was there space? Was it GOSH or UCLH? It seemed to take forever.

Then, suddenly, she was going. She was strapped into the transfer incubator. She was currently stable. Emma was still recovering from her traumatic labour. She needed further care before she could be discharged. My mother-in-law, Caroline, was coming to look after her while I was to go with Sophie in the ambulance. *See you at UCLH …*

◊

I cannot now remember if it was in the hospital, outside the building, or on arrival at UCLH, but I distinctly remember Mick, the paramedic/driver, congratulating me on having a baby daughter in a cheery and entirely authentic way. At face value this would seem like an insensitive or flippant comment. It wasn't. It was one of the nicest things that has ever been said to me, and at the most important time.

Firstly, it was said honestly and with genuine humanity – who doesn't take pride in the birth of their first child and the collective attention that affirms it? Much more importantly, it was the first positive thing we'd heard since Emma had gone into labour and was in such contrast to the cacophony and chaos of all the crises that had been unfolding since the moment of her birth.

It was a distant ray of sunlight in a stormy sky that served as a reminder that all storms pass. It affirmed that we had a daughter, that she was real, and she was precious. It gave her, if not agency, then significance. It's amazing how even small sentences, inadvertently spoken, can mean so much.

So, there we were. My first morning as a father. Leaving the hospital through the staff exit with my firstborn child in a mobile intensive care cot and an NTS entourage leading us to their ambulance.

I sat beside Sophie in the back. The medical team were sitting next to her, keeping an eye on her stats, and reading charts, as the ambulance swayed out and headed toward Central London. Blue lights on. Sirens wailing at junctions. In any other circumstance it would have been an enjoyable experience to bypass the perennial London traffic.

This was our home turf. The handsome whitewash stucco and yellow brick of the late-Victorian and early-Georgian architecture flitted by. The tube stations. The park. Familiar sights from Saturday walks. The London traffic grudgingly yielding to the siren. This experience, and subsequent experiences in hospital, have convinced me that where we are physically is not ever the same as where we are mentally.

What do I mean? I mean that I was in my home turf in our favourite part of London. Just outside the ambulance were normal people living their normal lives in a happy part of the world.

I was metres away, separated only by the thin aluminium walls of the ambulance. I was also a million miles away: like a desperate migrant on the wrong side of a barbed wire fence; like the homeless person on the streets of Mayfair, close to the homes of the super-rich. So close. So far.

There was a void so great it could not be filled. Flinging the doors open and leaping out would have made no difference to my reality, there in the ambulance. My dearest, already cherished, desperately sick daughter was there. A million miles away from where we had been just hours before.

My soul had become a black hole that swallowed all life's normality. Appetite, ambition and normal conscious thought was sucked into oblivion and replaced by a cold, dark, all-consuming fear.

They say your life changes fundamentally when you become a parent. Yes. Anyone who has had a seriously ill child also knows how life changes fundamentally when that happens. Now it had happened to us. There was no going back. Would we only carry loss and grief forward? Would we ever carry Sophie home back up this hill? This was my hellish journey down the Hampstead Road.

A new home: UCLH NICU

We arrived at University College London Hospital. The transfer team took us in through the A&E entrance and followed their well-trodden path to the NICU in the Elizabeth Garrett Anderson Wing. Hospital wards were a new experience for me. The white walls, the bright lights, the electromagnetic locked doors, the sinister smell of hand sanitiser. We eventually made it into the waiting room of the NICU, a place we would come to know well over the next few weeks. Our port in a storm.

Sophie was so ensconced in medical equipment that it was hard even to see her, let alone know how she was getting on. The transfer team became more business-like as they neared the end of their role.

All this had been a completely unreal experience, like those anxious, half-awake, half-asleep dreams you get with a fever. It was bizarre because my emotional state was confused. The fundamental emotions which bind a person to their newborn child were there, but we had never been able to hold her. I don't know if either of us had even touched her. As a result, I was chaperoning a little being who was both infinitely close to me and a complete stranger. Her identity was paper thin, like a spectre or ghost.

And then she was taken from me and I was asked to sit in the waiting room. Blue plastic chairs in rows. Medical information posters on walls. Sinks, soap dispensers, blue paper towels. Other parents. Conversations vaguely impinging on my consciousness. Not sinking in. A busy receptionist working at the computer and getting up to track down colleagues.

Sophie was wheeled off by the NTS team and a senior nurse into the ICU. I had to wait while they stabilised her in the nursery. I was alone. I had never felt so alone. The first day of being a father. No child. No wife. No ebullient friends or proud grandparents. No selfies or social media posts. Abjectly alone. Was this our fault? Did we deserve this? I'd give anything for her not to suffer.

When someone goes through a traumatic experience the adrenaline and passage of events can act as a protective barrier from the worst of the reality. I think the human brain is either incapable of taking it all in, or is cleverly designed to shield you from properly registering what is unfolding. What you really have to worry about is silence. Silence fills the space that was frenetic, and then the emotions hit. A great wave that builds and builds and then crashes down over you.

I could have been sitting there for minutes, it must have been closer to hours. I remember sobbing great racking sobs. The waiting room was now quite empty; it was early in the morning after all. I was oblivious. I'm sure there are words for how I felt: fear, grief, deep sadness, self-pity, tiredness; an emotional crash after going through a tricky labour with my dearest Emma and the resulting crisis; the dark birth suite, the doctors filing in, us thinking they were going to tell us we had lost her. And none of these.

My parental instincts kicked back in after a while. No one had come to find me. How was she? Was she alive? Where was she? I stood up in my distressed and spent state to ask. There didn't seem to be anyone there.

Eventually, a friendly, pretty, capable nurse came to see me. One of the countless angels in that building. I explained my situation. I think she brought me some tea. She explained they would take some time getting her set up in the hospital's incubator, and that they would be doing tests, and that the best thing for Sophie would be for them to be left to stabilise her.

She was kind and understanding. She knew I felt the need to do something to care for my baby, but that I had to accept this stage was out of my hands. The fundamental mismatch between the drive to care for your child and the medical reality of having a baby in the NICU, the fact you are so very out of control was, for me, one of the hardest things to accept about being a parent in NICU.

I was finally summoned into Room One, which we later learnt is reserved for the sickest babies. Sophie was in Cot Two. I didn't know then that this large room, its four strange incubator beds, hundreds of machines, wires and beeping chimes, was the very best place in the whole world for her to be, or that the staff were nothing short of medical miracle workers.

It was an alien environment. All this time Sophie had been under heavy sedation. An oscillating ventilator was hooked up to her, which gave off a loud rhythmic pumping sound. Wires and pipes were attached everywhere, and an EEG cap was on her head, monitoring her brain activity.

I was able to stand next to her and talk to her, not quite sure what to say. I probably told her that I loved her and that the doctors were doing everything they could to look after her. That her Daddy was with her and that Mummy would be there as soon as she could. I hope my words, my voice, were familiar to her and offered a modicum of reassurance.

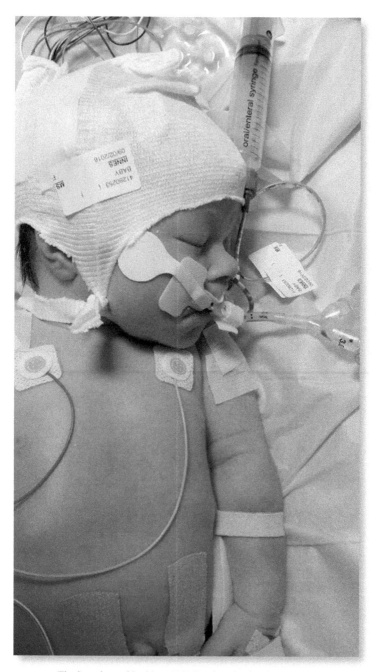

The first photo of Sophie at UCLH, taken the day she was born

Chapter Nine

Emma

I just want to get to UCLH. I want to be with her. I want to know what is happening. I don't want to be stuck in a small, clinical bereavement room by myself. I am not bereaved! I have a baby and I want to be with her.

I should be resting, even sleeping. I should be letting my body recuperate. Allowing it to start the long recovery process. But I'm not. I'm impatient.

Despite having only just given birth, I drag myself out of bed. I can't leave in a dressing gown so I fish some well-worn maternity clothes out of my bag and get dressed. I still have a big bump; I still look heavily pregnant. But my baby is no longer in the safety of my womb. She is out in a cold, bright world experiencing the most brutal introduction to life imaginable.

When she should have been being fed and cuddled and cooed over, she was being ventilated and intubated and sedated. Rather than the gentle, loving hand of her parents, the first things to touch her skin were needles and monitors and plasters. Her first experience of life was of near-death, of drowning, of not being able to breathe.

I have to get to her.

I make my way tentatively to the midwives' station in the corridor and ask to be discharged. I am sent back to my room to wait. Paperwork has to be completed. Discharge papers. There is an injection I need. Observations to be taken.

I don't care – I want to get to my baby! But I will have to be patient.

How can I possibly be patient when my baby is fighting for her life in a different hospital? I perch myself on the edge of the bed not looking remotely patient.

I receive an email from Dad, who is at home looking after my disabled brother, Edward, requesting a picture of Sophie and asking how much she weighs. I send him the one picture I have. A picture of her lying in her critical care cot with half her face obscured by a ventilator. I think she looks utterly gorgeous. He knows she is very unwell but it must be painful to see the reality. It isn't how newborn photos should look.

I'm also stunned by the question about her weight. Who cares? It's irrelevant. So trivial; such a normal question to ask in such abnormal circumstances. I assume my ancient grandmothers are insisting that Dad finds out the weight. That is the kind of thing old people like to know about babies. 'Oh, darling! How lovely! How much does the baby weigh?' I get it. I get that they probably don't have any concept of how sick she is. I understand that knowing what to ask in these circumstances, what to say, is difficult. I don't mind them asking. I know the answer to that question – she weighs eight pounds. It just seems odd to me.

◊

Into the room comes a cheery, if robot-like, promo woman. It beggars belief. She sets off on her spiel about which nappies I should use, which freebies she is going to give me, which free magazine she has for me. How can she be so insensitive? Can she not see I am in the bereavement room? Can she not see I don't have a baby? Can she not see how inappropriate this is? Nappies are the last thing on my mind. I am worried about whether my baby is still alive – I couldn't care less about the relative merits of Pampers versus Tesco own brand. Has she not realised that all of the mums with babies are on a ward? Surely she spends enough time in postnatal to know what the private rooms are used for?

I stare at her in disbelief unable to say anything. By this point, Mum has miraculously appeared and she throws her out.

'Can't you see she doesn't have a baby with her? Do you think this is appropriate right now? Please leave her alone.'

While Mum is with me, a midwife arrives and sets about trying to encourage me to start hand-expressing milk. It is vital, she says, to start encouraging milk production. If I don't do it, I won't be able to breastfeed. I am told to stimulate milk production as a feeding newborn would. I should use my thumb and forefinger to squeeze tiny quantities of colostrum (the first, antibody-rich milk) from my swollen breasts. If I don't, my body won't produce milk and my baby needs milk.

I'm not interested. It's all too much. I want to be left alone now. I'm not in the right frame of mind for trying to master this new skill. It feels irrelevant. Sophie is probably going to die. Why do I need to worry about breastfeeding a baby who can't breathe, let alone feed? I have more important things to worry about. I'll deal with this later, if necessary. I'm too tired.

However, Mum and the midwife are having none of it. They insist that I commit to the process. They ensure that I keep trying to master hand-expressing the milk. They tell me it is important. I find it awkward and embarrassing.

◊

I came to be extremely glad that Mum and the midwife had insisted I attempt the hand-expressing. Otherwise, I wouldn't have been able to breastfeed Sophie. In the end, I fed her this way for a year. A very precious year.

◊

Mum proceeds to chivvy the midwives in her usual business-like fashion. She understands that I need to be with Sophie and does everything she can to ensure I get to UCLH as quickly as possible. She's on a mission to look after her daughter. I've seen her in this state many times and this mood means business!

Eventually, with much urging – 'Come on! She needs to be with her baby!' – progress is made: I'm given my injection; I'm discharged around lunchtime. It's a relief to let Mum be my advocate, to let her be in charge. I need someone else to take control.

We slowly make our way out of the hospital, Mum insists I get some lunch from the hospital shop on the way. Left to my own devices, I'd skip lunch. I'm not interested. Not hungry. Exclusively focused on getting to Sophie. But Mum is right. I must have expended a huge amount of energy during the labour and I need to eat. I need to remember what my body has been through and to look after it. I'm no use to Sophie if I'm ill too.

Jamie has sent me a brief message saying that Sophie is allowed to have a small teddy in her incubator. For comfort. To cuddle next to her. To give her medicalised bed a more homely feel. I don't have any soft toys in the hospital bag. I just know, in my mind, that if the doctors say she can have a teddy, then she must have one. We go into the WHSmith on the ground floor of the hospital to look for a teddy. Choices are seriously limited. Most are huge. Clearly not appropriate for an incubator. There's only one option. A small blue creature. Something like a cross between a cow and a hippo. He becomes known affectionately as Blue Cow.

Outside, Mum and I hail the first black cab we see and ask to be taken to UCLH. The cab driver must

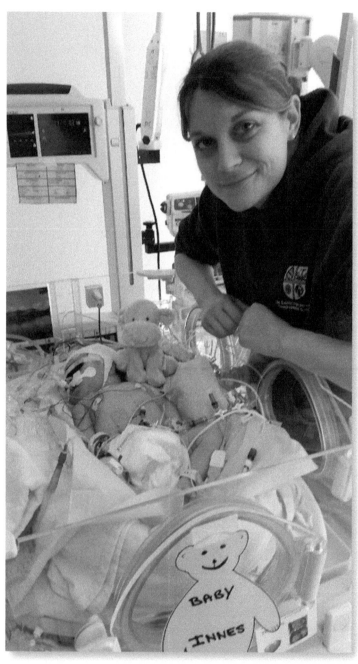

Emma with a two-day-old Sophie, Blue Cow
standing to attention on her shoulder

wonder what our story is. He must wonder why we're hopping from one hospital to another. Why we look so pale and upset. I'm still clutching my hospital bag full of newborn nappies and clothes, as yet untouched.

Jamie's messaged me with details of how to find them. He and Sophie are in the NICU in the Elizabeth Garrett Anderson Wing at UCLH.

◊

Jamie

Things became much easier for me when Emma arrived at lunchtime. Never had I loved my wife so much or been prouder of her. There she was, having just given birth for the first time and without painkillers.

She'd had a significant episiotomy and lost a good deal of blood. She was battered and bruised by the labour and had gone through what must be one of the hardest things for a mother – her baby had nearly died, was terribly sick, and she'd not been able to hold her. Yet there she was. On her feet. Calm, dignified, clearly moved by the whole experience but completely composed. Loving and unbroken. Practical and to the point.

We embraced as a thousand feelings were expressed in one touch. She said it will be as it will be. What a girl. I couldn't have gone through the following weeks without her. Her strength was inspirational. It's a good thing Sophie has her mother's stoicism, because over the next ten days she was really going to need it.

Part Two
The Last Chance
Ventilator

February Nine

The taxi drops Mum and me at the entrance to the Elizabeth Garrett Anderson Unit, on a side street behind the main UCLH building.

Following the directions in Jamie's text, we make our way through the foyer and up the lift, past Maternity and Gynaecology, to the Neonatal Unit. This will become a well-trodden path for us: traversing lifts; navigating endless hospital corridors; being buzzed in.

We wait for the receptionist to let us in. The door opens into the waiting room. To our left is the reception desk, to our right, a consultation room and the milk expressing room.

The walls are lined with blue plastic chairs and lockers for parents to keep their belongings in. Immediately in front of us is a corridor, The Corridor, guarded by a conspicuous sink complete with hospital-grade soap, hand sanitiser, blue paper towels and a foot-pedal-operated bin that clanks when it closes.

Because we're new to this place, we have to be taught the rules. This job falls to the receptionist. She explains to Mum and me that we must put our coats and bags in a locker – that we mustn't take anything onto the unit to reduce the infection risk. We must remove all rings, watches and bracelets – again, to reduce the risk of infection. She shows us how to wash our hands properly. They must be wetted, scrubbed with soap, rinsed, dried on a paper towel and then rubbed with hand sanitiser. We must go through this whole routine every time we enter The Corridor.

The Corridor, the unit proper, with eight four-bed nurseries. Rooms One and Two are intensive care, Rooms Three and Four are high dependency, the rest are special care. You want to be in the highest number room possible. You want to work your way along the corridor to special care as your baby gets better. That's the aim.

We're shown to Room One. The worst place to be. And yet, also the best place to be. The worst place to be in that it is reserved for the four sickest babies on the unit. But the best place to be, if you are unlucky enough to need to be there. World-class neonatal care is offered in this room by highly skilled professionals. Some of the best neonatologists in the world work in this room. If your baby needs intensive care, this is the place to be.

Anyway, here we are. Sophie isn't just in intensive care, she's in the most intensive room of the ICU of a leading London hospital. At this moment, she's one of the sickest babies in the capital.

◊

In retrospect, we feel incredibly lucky that Sophie was given a cot in Room One of the UCLH NICU. It's so fortunate that she was born near to such an amazing facility, that they had space for her, and that they agreed to take her at the crack of dawn. They could so easily have been full. They could have said no. They could have deemed her beyond help.

We are so lucky that we have the NHS to pick up the pieces in catastrophes like this. That we didn't have to spend a second worrying about the mind-blowing cost of her care. That in our moment of need everything was just organised for us – the NHS emergency cogs whirring into action and Sophie being rescued from imminent death, without us doing anything.

◊

When we reach Room One, we're told that before entering the nursery we will need to go through the hand washing routine again. Every time we enter the unit, and every time we enter a nursery on the unit. If we pop out to get a glass of water or a sandwich, we must do it again. If we go to the loo we must wash our hands in the bathroom, then again to re-enter The Corridor, and again to enter the nursery. If we go out into the corridor to answer the phone, we must wash our hands again before returning to the nursery. So it goes on.

◊

We both struggled with the constant use of powerful soaps and hand sanitisers in the NICU, but I suffered particularly. My hands were already dry at the end of pregnancy and the end of the winter. After a few days on NICU they were raw, red, cracked and bleeding.

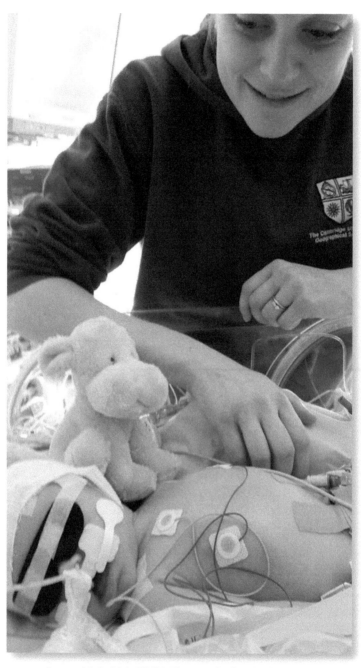

Emma with Sophie in NICU. The cap on her head holds the EEG sensors in place; earplugs and eye mask prevent overstimulation; Blue Cow stands to attention on her shoulder

Putting the hand sanitiser on was agony. Just moving my fingers became uncomfortable as the cracked skin stretched and broke further. My clothes had little spots of blood on them from where my hands had bled as I got dressed. They were the first visible manifestation of the physical and emotional strain we were under.

◊

Room One has four cots in it, one in each corner. Sophie is in Cot Two, in the back-left corner. Her companions for most of her time in this room will be Henry, born at twenty-three weeks gestation, in the front-left corner, and Finn, delivered at twenty-four weeks gestation, in the back-right corner. The final cot is empty.

I'm shown to Sophie's cot. By the window. An incubator surrounded by a mind-blowing array of machines and wires with a little desk at one end. Every cot has a desk and stool at the end of it. Because every baby in the ICU receives one-to-one nursing. I can't believe it when I'm told that, 24/7, there will be an intensive care nurse whose sole purpose during her shift will be to look after Sophie. The desk at the end of Sophie's incubator is the nurse's desk. That is where she will spend her shift, looking after my baby constantly for twelve hours straight.

I feel safe in the knowledge that Sophie is being so well cared for. I almost feel inadequate. These nurses are clearly better placed to be changing her nappy, giving her her milk and looking after her than I am. They are highly trained professionals. I have never looked after a baby for a single moment in my entire life. I'm glad, in a way, that it is them caring for her rather than me.

◊

The level of care is unbelievable. The cost of it impossible to fathom. The amount of time, expertise and equipment that is being employed in a bid to save our little girl is incredible. What the NHS can offer, what society collectively provides for people in desperate need, is staggering. All for one tiny baby no one yet knew. All of this to fight for her. It is truly humbling.

◊

Sophie is lying in her incubator, sedated and immobilised by muscle-paralysing medication, surrounded by machinery and sporting a pair of vast, orange earplugs and an eye mask to prevent her being overstimulated by the busy environment. She's hooked up to an oscillating ventilator. Behind her are two banks of shunts, eight shunts in total, automatically administering her medication day and night through a network of wires. She has a cap on her head covering numerous EEG sensors monitoring her brain activity, and she is surrounded by computers. Computers tracking her brain activity, showing her vital signs, registering her temperature. She's lying on pads of cool water to keep her body temperature at thirty-three degrees. She has a canister of nitric oxide to her left, to help open her blood vessels and reduce the blood pressure in her lungs. To her right is a little hospital stool for a parent to perch on. At her feet is the nurses' station. There are more gadgets and machines around her but I have no idea what they do.

Sophie is on industrial quantities of antibiotics, morphine, synthetic hormones and much more. She's on full life support. The maximum support the UCLH NICU can offer a baby. The only way she could be given more support would be for her to be transferred to GOSH for heart-lung bypass.

She's on the rarely wheeled out oscillating ventilator. The so-called Last Chance Ventilator. The ventilator they use when nothing else is sufficient. One of the consultants cheerfully tells me that he has no idea why it works. He just knows it does.

The oscillating ventilator, or high-frequency ventilator, makes a constant throbbing sound as it pulses away, delivering very small breaths very rapidly. Tick-a-tick-a-tick-a-tick. All day and all night. Relentlessly. Keeping her alive. Keeping her oxygenated. It doesn't create a normal breathing action. Sophie's bare chest isn't rising and falling as a chest should. It's vibrating. There's no reassuring, rhythmic rise and fall as she breathes; her chest is shuddering constantly. Fluttering away up to 900 times a minute.

I'll never forget the noise of that machine. It was the soundtrack to Sophie's time in intensive care. Our constant companion as we sat beside her. Reassuring in its constant rhythm.

◊

When I reach Sophie's side, the nurse looking after her asks me if I know what's happening. I tell her the few details I know. She fills me in.

She starts by saying: 'She is in intensive care.'

She then goes on to explain what's wrong with her and what care she's receiving. She tells us that the doctors are watching her brain activity very closely, looking for any sign of fits. For any sign that she has severe brain damage. Fits are what they are concerned about. If she has a fit, it will suggest significant brain damage. She will be hooked up to the EEG machine constantly for seventy-two hours. Three days of constant brain activity monitoring to establish if she will have lifelong disabilities resulting from oxygen starvation.

I'm not worrying about the possibility of severe brain damage, or of disability. I'm too shocked to think much at all, to take it all in. All of my energy is reserved for willing her to survive.

◊

We came to learn that your priorities change as your baby goes through their journey in the NICU. When they are desperately sick all that matters to you is that they live. At that point, you would accept any degree of disability in return for being able to keep your baby. It's only as they start to improve, only once their life is no longer in immediate danger, that you start to worry about the long-term prognosis.

Once you know they will live, you start to worry about severe disability or long-term health problems. Once it becomes clear that they don't have either of these, the possibility of minor disabilities starts to bother you. You go from being more than happy to accept catastrophic brain damage in return for life, to worrying about the tiny things most parents worry about – are they slightly later to smile than average, are they gaining weight fast enough, do they make eye contact properly? Your perspective changes as the severity of their situation changes.

◊

The nurse looking after Sophie also goes through the housekeeping. She shows us the drawer in the desk where we can store a few things. She suggests maybe a few books to read to Sophie, the diary Jamie is just starting and a small teddy bear. She also tells us that all babies on the unit are allowed visits from their parents and a maximum of four other, named individuals – usually the grandparents. No one else is allowed to visit to reduce the risk of infection. We're asked to write down the names of the other people we would like to be allowed in. We name my parents, Paul and Caroline, Jamie's mum, Mary, and Jamie's sister, Natalie.

Mum and I stand beside her taking it all in. This is Mum's first glimpse of her granddaughter. Of a baby fighting for her life, surrounded by machines, testing medical science to its limits. If she deteriorates further … I don't know. I think she will die.

◊

Mary and Natalie arrive during the afternoon. Jamie said calling them was difficult and upsetting. He felt that telling someone what had happened somehow made it seem even more real. Only two visitors were allowed by Sophie's incubator at any one time so the rest had to remain in the waiting room.

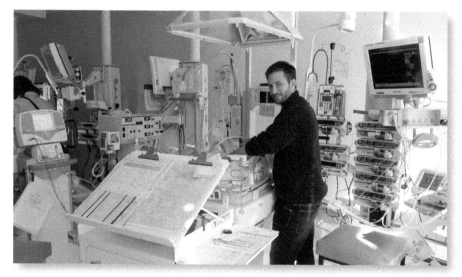

*Jamie with Sophie in NICU; all the medical equipment
in the photo is connected to her*

Emma's mum, Caroline, with Sophie in NICU

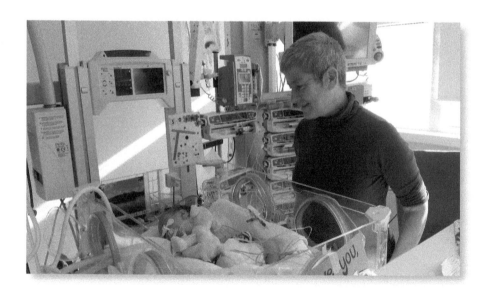

My recollections of that afternoon are very sketchy. I don't remember much about it at all. I recollect Mary asking us if we had a name for her.

I looked at Jamie as if to say: 'Sophie? Happy? Are you still sure? Is that definitely what we're going with? Shall we tell them?'

He nodded at me. Our decision from the Royal Free still stood.

It was a huge decision. In other circumstances we might have mulled it over for longer. At that moment, it didn't seem particularly important. We didn't have the energy to consider it further and we've not regretted it for a second. It was a decision made in haste, in desperate circumstances when we were in no fit state to be making important decisions. But I think it was a good decision.

Standing by the blue chairs in the waiting room we said: 'Sophie. We're calling her Sophie.'

It should have been a big reveal. A big moment. But it wasn't. Bigger things were happening. We were just glad to be able to refer to her by name.

We were glad, too, to have our family around us, although these were not the circumstances in which we had imagined introducing them to our baby. There was no joy or excitement. No congratulations. Worry and upset were written across everyone's face. We almost felt as though we had let them down. They must have been looking forward to meeting and holding the new baby. This wasn't how it was supposed to be. It was all wrong. It was intensely traumatic in the moment but, also, opened up huge uncertainty for the future. Did this baby have a future and, if so, what would her life be like?

◊

A friendly, young nurse called Sapphire comes to find me. She explains that she helps the new mums on the unit establish their breastfeeding routines. The unit is very keen that as many babies as possible are fed their mother's breastmilk.

Breastmilk, particularly the colostrum that is produced in the few days after giving birth, is extremely high in antibodies. Vital extra defence for vulnerable new babies. A parting gift from the mother.

She tells me that Sophie isn't currently able to tolerate very much milk at all. She is too sick. But she says the nurse looking after her will give her as much as she can manage and that she will benefit hugely from it.

Sapphire then introduces me to the Milk Expressing Room – The Dairy, as I come to know it. It's a small room off the waiting room, with a few chairs, a long table along the back wall and a handful of electric breast pumps. A row of mums sit expressing milk. I will become familiar with this exceptionally bizarre social set up but, for now, it's all new to me.

Sapphire kindly and sensitively shows me where the room is, how to use the machines, how to disinfect them before using them and how to label any bottles of milk I produce. She tells me that all milk I manage to express should be labelled with the time and date and my baby's name, and given to the nurse looking after her. It will then either be fed directly through Sophie's feeding tube, or frozen for when she needs it.

Sapphire also tells me that to ensure a good supply of milk, I must express milk from each breast at least every three hours. If I don't, the milk won't come in properly and I won't produce enough.

The quantity of milk a mother produces in the first couple of days of her baby's life is so small that Sapphire gives me a five-millilitre syringe and shows me how to hand-express tiny quantities of colostrum. Harvesting whole bottles of milk using the machines will have to wait for a few days. For now, just a few millilitres is an achievement to be proud of.

Sapphire is understanding and experienced but it is an uncomfortable experience. Embarrassing and awkward. But it has to be done. There's no other choice. The NICU staff are clear that unless there is a very good excuse, all mums should express milk because it is the best, most nutritious sustenance for very sick or very small babies. It is particularly important for premature babies as their immature guts are often unable to digest formula milk.

◊

Early in the evening of Sophie's first day, someone comes to tell me they've found me a bed in the building if I want to stay overnight. I suspect they worked hard to do that. It's so kind of them and I genuinely appreciate the offer. But it doesn't mean I can stay next to Sophie; the bed isn't even in the neonatal part of the building. I just want to go home. Home to our bed. Home to familiarity. To a clean shower, clean clothes, some decent food. To normality.

There is nothing we can do for Sophie. She is sedated, she doesn't know we are there, we can't offer her anything that the wonderful nurses and doctors aren't already providing. It's them she needs right now and we trust them entirely. Also, we've been up for thirty-six hours and counting. So, at about seven in the evening, we leave the hospital and take a taxi back up the hill to home.

We have to walk out of the hospital without our new baby. We have to trust the doctors and nurses to look after her in our absence. And trust them we do.

◊

It's heart-breaking to leave her there, by herself. It feels all wrong. And yet it doesn't. It would probably feel even more surreal arriving home with a baby. I'm used to not having a baby with me. Having a baby to take home would be far more unfamiliar.

And there is the empty Moses basket, the unused pile of baby clothes … all as it was yesterday. Yet, everything has changed. Yesterday it was right that the Moses basket was empty. Now, it's all wrong. She should be sleeping peacefully, dressed in a tiny new outfit. But she isn't. She's lying, naked but for a nappy, in an incubator. Worst of all, she isn't with us, where she should be.

We eat, shower and change, largely in silence. Together but alone with our thoughts. We're exhausted. We don't know what to say. During crises I tend to become detached and practical, I suppose it is my coping mechanism. Doing what I have to do unemotionally protects me. Jamie finds this reassuring and he is more emotional so leans on me for support.

Before I can collapse into bed, I have to set up my new, and as yet unused, breast pump, for the three-hour expressing rule applies day and night. Exhausted as I am, I will have to set an alarm to wake me up every three hours to express more tiny quantities of colostrum. I'll then have to label them, put them in the fridge and give them to the nurse in the morning. I don't have a baby with me. I don't have a baby to look after. But I still have to get up throughout the night to provide milk. It's a cruel irony. I feel I should at least be spared the broken nights. That should be the one, tiny benefit of the situation. But, no, the sleep deprivation has well and truly started.

We have been given a phone number for Room One. At any time of the day or night we can call it and get directly through to the nurse looking after Sophie. We can call for an update on her condition or just for reassurance. We discuss whether to call. We don't want to disturb the nurse when she's busy looking after Sophie, but we want to know. There's also an element of wanting to look like diligent parents. Surely diligent, loving parents would check up on their daughter. We agree that we'll call just before going to bed and on waking tomorrow.

It's difficult. What if the call brings bad news? We tiptoe around the issue of who will make the call. In the end, Jamie admits he's not up to it. He can't face any more bad news. So I call, happy to be able to take one tiny burden off his shoulders. I have butterflies. I am nervous. Jamie leaves the room, not wanting to hear what is said.

Me: 'Hi, my name's Emma. I'm Sophie's mum. I was wondering if you could give me an update on how she's doing.'

Nurse: 'Of course! Don't worry. She's stable. She's fine. She's just as she was when you left. We'll look after her tonight – you get some sleep.'

Me: 'Thank you so much. See you tomorrow.'

Nurse: 'Yes. See you tomorrow.

February Ten

*I*t's the day after Sophie was born. We wake up to our new reality, to a new routine. We drag ourselves out of bed, I express more milk and we call to find out how she's been overnight. Then we get dressed, force down some breakfast, collect the night's milk from the fridge, and catch a taxi to the NICU.

The journey is fraught with anxiety. What will we find when we arrive? Even though we'd called first thing in the morning, it's nerve-wracking. We know her condition can change extremely fast.

When we walk into the waiting room, I'm hit once again by the smell of hospital cleaning products, hospital soap and hand sanitiser. Once I've been inside for a few minutes, I stop noticing it.

There is a very distinctive smell to NHS soap. To this day, if I smell that soap, I am immediately transported back to the NICU. Every time I come across it in the GP surgery, I feel slightly sick. That smell will forever be linked with Sophie's time in intensive care. The faintest waft of it and for a moment I am at the hospital sink in Room One.

◊

The main event of the morning on the NICU is the ward round, when the consultants go to each baby in turn, discuss their progress and update their families. All the parents aim to be there for the ward round. The mums dread missing it by being in The Dairy at just the wrong moment. It is your chance to get a full update on how your baby is doing and to ask any questions. You hang on the doctor's every word, desperate for them to offer hope, dreading more bad news. Everything depends on what they say. They can reassure you that your baby is improving, that they will live. Or they can break the news that they are worried about your precious child – that they have deteriorated, that they aren't making the expected progress, that they have concerning symptoms. The ward round is vital. It can determine whether you have a positive day or a terrible one. It can give you optimism or dash all hope.

The parents on the unit linger close to their babies all morning waiting for the consultants to arrive, for fear of missing them. Rumours spread about when they will arrive, whether the round is running late, where on the ward they currently are. Parents debate how long it will be before the doctors enter the room.

Eventually, mid-morning, the door of Room One opens and in walks the consultant and his entourage. He comes over to our corner of the room and introduces himself as Sophie's consultant, Dr Giles Kendall.

Dr Kendall. He's to become a huge figure in our lives. He's responsible for Sophie's care. He decides how to treat her. He's the one who can tell us how she's doing, whether she has a chance at life and what her long-term prognosis is. He holds everything that matters to us in his hands.

Despite the rigours of his job, Dr Kendall is youthful. He looks younger than his years and his experience. He conveys an infectious positivity and cheerfulness. He's kind and calm and optimistic, while also being astoundingly clever, highly skilled and knowledgeable. He is clearly passionate about what he does. Despite the hugely long hours he works, and the traumas he witnesses on a daily basis, never once did I see him look weary, downbeat or harassed.

He tells us that Sophie has had a decent night and that she's stable. That she has possibly even improved slightly and he is happy with her progress. He explains that if all goes to plan, she will be in intensive care for at least a week, on the ventilator, to give her lungs a chance to recover. He says she still requires a huge amount of support but that he hopes to gradually wean her off it altogether.

Dr Kendall gives us a far greater sense of hope than we had at the Royal Free. However, he is also realistic. He admits that even if she does really well, she will need to be in hospital for weeks because it will take a long time for her lungs to recover fully. He thinks she will struggle to remain oxygenated while feeding.

We are delighted with this update. Here is someone talking about recovery. He's worrying about things like feeding. At this point, we don't care how long she has to stay in hospital. All that matters is that she lives. We would have been ecstatic just to be able to hold her, to cuddle her, to dress her. If that has to be in hospital, that's fine. All that matters is to get to be parents to our baby.

As things stand, she is a day old and we haven't held her. We haven't had a chance to cuddle her. We can rest a hand on any tiny part of her that isn't covered with wires but that's the only physical contact we can have with her. The idea of being able to hold her is magical. But it will have to wait for at least a week. There's no guarantee we will ever get there.

◊

Just after our second child, George, was born, a relative was giving me detailed instructions on how to ensure one is discharged from the postnatal ward as quickly as possible. On how I should put pressure on the midwives to have the newborn checks carried out promptly so I could get home within the day. I was astonished. I couldn't believe he thought it mattered and I was hurt that he thought I didn't know what it was like to have a baby. That somehow my experience with Sophie didn't count as experience with a newborn.

I was completely relaxed about whether I was discharged on the day of the birth, or the following day. I felt so lucky that I had a healthy baby in my arms nothing else mattered. I couldn't believe that, second time round, I had just given birth and I actually had a baby with me. A baby to cuddle and feed and coo over. The last thing I was going to do was to pester busy NHS midwives to attend to me and my healthy baby more rapidly. I was well aware that they had more important things to do.

Our experience with Sophie was very good for giving us perspective.

◊

After updating us on Sophie's care, Dr Kendall moves on to another vital factor. Brain damage. He tells us that, miraculously, despite a significant period of oxygen deprivation, she's showing no signs of severe brain damage. She hasn't had any fits and her EEG shows her brain activity to be essentially normal.

This is huge. It doesn't rule out some degree of damage but it strongly suggests she doesn't have catastrophic brain damage. It means that, if she can be kept alive long enough for her lungs to recover, she has a future and that it could, possibly, be a healthy one.

Leaving us feeling deeply reassured and more hopeful about Sophie than before, Dr Kendall moves on to the next cot. Sophie's nurse then gives Jamie and me a pair of headphones each to wear while the doctors discuss the other babies in the room. All parents are asked to wear noise-cancelling headphones if they remain in the nursery while the doctors are discussing one of the other babies. It's a way of ensuring patient confidentiality without having to repeatedly ask parents to leave their baby.

◊

During the afternoon, having had a positive morning, we start to settle into life on the NICU. We know we are going to be here for a long time so we have to settle into a routine. I'm busy with regular trips to The Dairy to express more tiny quantities of colostrum.

Meanwhile, Jamie and Natalie follow the nurse's advice to read to Sophie. Jamie's diary mentions that Natalie read *Elmer the Elephant* and that he read *Goodnight Moon*. We took to reading to her every day. My dad read her *The BFG*, we all read from a collection of AA Milne poems. It was a strange and slightly uncomfortable experience. Reading to an unconscious baby seems counterintuitive. Like talking to yourself. We felt self-conscious doing it. But, it was one of the very few things we could do for her and the doctors and nurses strongly encouraged it. They said babies found the sound of their parents' voices reassuring, familiar from their time in the womb. Supposedly, it calmed them. We were happy to do anything we could – glad to have a role.

Dad was probably the one most comfortable doing this. He knew that talking to her was encouraged so he read to her, but he also chatted away happily without a book. One quiet afternoon in the NICU he was left in charge while I was in The Dairy and Jamie was getting some lunch. He used the opportunity to explain to her, in detail, the causes and effects of the 1992 recession …

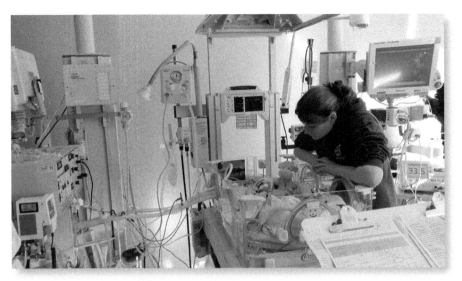

Emma with Sophie in the UCLH NICU

Natalie reading poems to Sophie the day after she was born

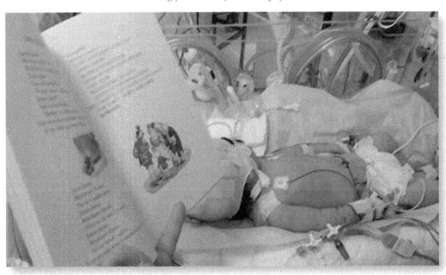

February Eleven

When we call the nursery in the morning, the news is less positive. Sophie has been very unstable overnight and she's developed another infection. The doctors have had to increase the amount of oxygen she's being given. This is not unexpected, but it is a setback. More bad news just as we have started to hope. It's an unwelcome reminder of just how sick she still is and the precariousness of her situation.

Jamie heads to the hospital first thing and by the time he arrives Sophie is stable again and it's back to business as usual in Room One. But it has shaken us. Taught us not to take anything for granted. That just because she has one good day, it doesn't mean that she will have another. That she's on a very bumpy journey.

Jamie's diary

'Daddy came extra early today to see me. He said that he misses me so much it hurts when he's not here, but that he falls in love each time he sees me.

'He read to me from *The BFG*, which was funny because he did a silly voice for the giant.

'He's very sweet but I can tell that he's sad because I know all he wants to hear is that the doctors think I'm getting better.

'He loves me very much because he squeezes my foot and pats my head in a friendly way.'

◊

I couldn't go with Jamie to the hospital as I have to stay at home for a visit from the midwife. A home visit that should be for me and Sophie. Instead, it's just for me.

The midwife has been briefed in advance as to my situation. When she arrives she asks awkwardly how Sophie's doing. I explain briefly, but I'm impatient with being a patient. I want to get to the hospital to be with Sophie. To hear how she is now. To see if she's stable again. To spend as much time as possible with her while I can. As soon as the midwife leaves, I head straight to the hospital.

◊

Jamie's diary

'Mummy, Daddy and Granny Mary spent lots of time with me today.

'Mummy and Daddy are going to paint my feet so they can get my footprints. How silly of them!'

'Daddy made such a mess with the purple ink that he had to give my foot its first bath.

'Mummy was very happy when she saw my hand and foot prints. She started crying because she thought they were beautiful.'

◊

Initially, I'd been uninterested in the idea of the footprints. Jamie was insistent, though. He was keen to do them as soon as possible. As soon as there was a quiet moment, when we wouldn't be in the way of the nurses. There was a sense of urgency about it for him. I was aware that he wanted to do them while he could because he feared he might not have much time.

◊

Having been very unstable during the night, the increased oxygen and a hefty dose of antibiotics have stabilised Sophie and she is making another tentative step forward.

Jamie's diary

'The doctors told Mummy and Daddy that I seem to be doing exactly what I should be.
'They told them all they should do is love me, touch me and talk to me. This made me very happy!'

◊

In the evening I send my Godmother an email:

'Sophie looks really strong and well on the outside so it's hard to believe she's so sick.
'In the bed next to her is a baby who was born at twenty-three weeks weighing five hundred grams. In most hospitals he was so premature his birth

would've been considered a miscarriage. He's just unbelievably tiny and Sophie looks enormous and strong as an ox next to him. I think I'm only just starting to realise the significance of the fact she's in a room with such obviously sick babies – not only is she in Intensive Care at a specialist central London hospital, she's also in the highest dependency room that Intensive Care Unit has. Poor little thing.'

Sophie's companions in Room One are two extremely premature babies. The first, Finn, weighs one pound ten, and the other only one pound one. Sophie looks huge next to them. Like a different species. You look at her and can't understand why she's there. Unlike her roommates, she doesn't look as though she should be. It is almost embarrassing. We feel like intruders. We aren't part of the club. We are in a different boat to the other parents in the room. Our baby's situation is completely different.

Finn's mum, Harriet, told me later that she was jealous of us. She even admitted to resenting us because in her world – at that time, a world of prematurity – all that mattered was size. I can understand that. She would have given anything for Finn to have been born at full-term like Sophie. Yet, as she acknowledged later, there was nothing enviable about Sophie's situation at that time. She was battling numerous life-threatening conditions at once. Her life still hung in the balance just as much as did those of Finn and Henry. The threat of brain damage still lingered over her. Neither her survival nor her long-term prognosis could be guaranteed.

◊

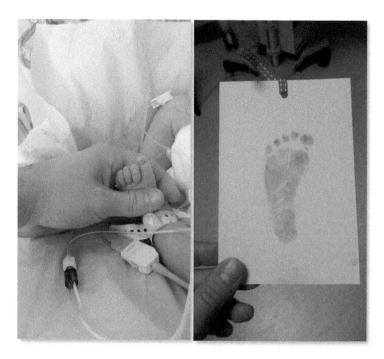

Taking a print of Sophie's foot when she was two days old and in NICU

Jamie's diary entry from February 14, 2016

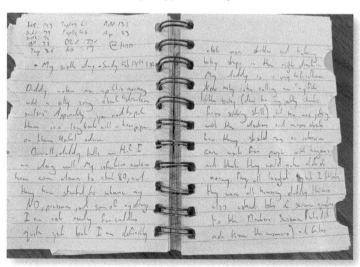

My little brother, Edward, who is three years younger than me, has Down's Syndrome. He is getting very cross because he has been looking forward to his niece's birth for months and is desperate to meet her. He is anxious to take up his role as 'awesome uncle'. But he can't because visiting rules in the NICU are so strict. Jamie and I promise him that as soon as it is possible, he will be the first person to visit her. The first to have a cuddle with her. This seems to satisfy him for the time being.

Edward has given me a different perspective on disability. It is, of course, not what I would want for my child. However, I'm not afraid of it because it isn't unfamiliar. I know from my own experience that a child with disabilities is just as much an integral, and loved, part of a family as any other child.

As we grew up, Edward was just Edward – my cheeky little brother. The fact he had Down's Syndrome wasn't relevant to family life on a day-to-day basis. He was – is – the heart and soul of the family and everyone adores him.

So, I know that if Sophie has disabilities resulting from the brain damage, we will love her just as much, and she'll be just as special to us as any child. I know that she'll still be a perfect addition to our family and that she'll still lead a fulfilling and rewarding life.

However, one thing sits uncomfortably with me. It's not difficult for me to accept Edward's disability because he is as he was always going to be from the moment of his conception. He's a perfect version of Edward. In contrast, if Sophie has brain damage she will not be how

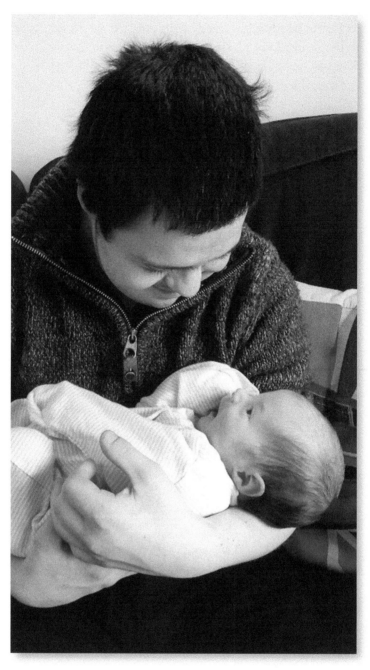

Edward finally takes up his role as 'awesome uncle' after Sophie leaves hospital

she was intended to be. She could have been different. Things could've been done that might have prevented the disability. She'll be a damaged version of what she might have been. That, I'd find much harder to live with. There would be guilt and questions. The thought that it might have been possible to prevent the disability in a way that it could, and should, never have been prevented in Edward. I know I'd be constantly thinking about the 'what-ifs', whereas this has never been the case with Edward.

February Twelve

We enter the unit to nothing but good news. Sophie's stable and has been all night. The doctors are gradually warming her up to a normal temperature. She has nearly completed her three days of cooling and it's hoped that she will start to recover more rapidly now. The cooling protected her brain, but it also put her into a kind of suspended animation that slowed her overall improvement. The doctors have now done what they can for her brain, so it's time to start trying to resurrect the rest of her body.

As part of this process, they reduce her sedation and take her off the drugs that have been paralysing her muscles. We see her move for the first time! At last, she can wriggle around a little, like a real baby.

Jamie and I sit beside her, watching. Desperate to see her move all of her limbs. Desperate to be reassured that she can move her whole body. Any movement seems like normality to us. In reality, this is far from the case. She's still on huge quantities of medication and is, anyway, too unwell to manage more than little wriggles.

While it is good for her to be able to move a little bit, she can't be allowed to do so much because she might dislodge her ventilator. Something as simple as shifting

Sophie into a different position, to keep her comfortable and prevent sores, requires a whole team of specialists. It also requires moving the ventilator and, to do that, she has to be briefly disconnected from the very thing that is keeping her alive.

As Jamie and I sit staring at Sophie, studying her every wriggle, the door opens. In come a group of doctors and nurses with a new baby to install. Finn. He has just been delivered at twenty-four weeks gestation, weighing one pound ten. He must only be minutes old. He was born in the UCLH Maternity Department which adjoins the NICU. The neonatologists from the unit were present at his birth, ready to stabilise him and rush him straight down the corridor to the waiting incubator in Room One.

The usually calm and measured atmosphere of Room One immediately changes. The room is suddenly busy and crowded. A calm and professional buzz, but intense activity as the doctors fight to stabilise Finn. To get him set up in his incubator, opposite Sophie.

All the attention in the room is on the new admission, so in our corner we focus on Sophie. We are there but not involved. We are spectators to a medical emergency, but spectators who don't want to be watching. We focus on Sophie because Finn and his family deserve privacy, not an audience, and the doctors need space to concentrate on getting this tiny, tiny baby safely installed.

After an hour or so, everything calms down. Finn is as stable in his incubator as the doctors can make him and everything in the room returns to normal. At this point,

Finn's parents are allowed to come and see him. Danny and Harriet. They become friends. They are like us. We are brothers in arms. They are also new young parents unexpectedly thrown into the NICU with a desperately ill first child. We discover later we have various mutual friends.

I really feel for them. We were in their position three days ago. New to the unit and the room. New to life on the NICU and new to parenthood. Trying to get our heads around what is wrong with our babies and what treatment they are receiving. Getting to know the doctors and nurses. Starting to get the hang of this new but very strange normal.

When you see new arrivals on the unit it is easy to focus on the baby and to forget that the mother has just given birth. Not only is she looking at her child in intensive care, she has just gone through the rigours of labour. She should be recuperating. Yet there she is, in an ICU, perched on an uncomfortable stool so that she's high enough to see her baby in the incubator. I know all too well that sitting on a stool when you've just had an episiotomy stitched up is not a comfortable experience. I understand Harriet's physical pain. I am experiencing it too.

We say hello to each other. Sophie and Finn are only six feet apart. This room is the whole world to all of us now. We know we'll be spending a lot of time next to them over the following days, maybe weeks. A lot of extremely difficult and emotional time. It is a strangely intense start to a new friendship.

Danny explains their story to us. Harriet went into labour at twenty-three weeks, the night before their wedding. Danny and many of the guests were in the hotel, ready for the ceremony the following day. A hotel porter had to drive him to the hospital to join Harriet as he was the only person sober enough! On the way they had been pulled over for speeding but when Danny explained the situation, the police drove him the rest of the way. The wedding was hastily called off. Harriet was initially told she was having a miscarriage. Eventually, doctors and paramedics were persuaded to give Finn a chance and she was transferred to UCLH where the delivery was delayed for a week. Now, here they are, in the NICU, with an extremely preterm baby.

Danny gives a half-hearted grin and says: 'Currently, I'm on honeymoon in Mauritius ...'

◊

After Sophie left UCLH, we thought a lot about Finn. We had got to know Danny and Harriet and felt a kinship with them. We wanted to get in touch to find out how he was doing. We knew that around the time we left the unit, Finn was transferred to GOSH, still desperately sick, needing surgery on his gut. We didn't know whether he had survived.

We frequently thought about messaging Harriet but we felt guilty that we were home with our baby. We were worried that Finn might have died and we knew that, even if he was still fighting, he would have a long road ahead of him in intensive care. We thought Harriet and Danny might not want to hear from us as we had reached the end of our NICU journey. As a result, we didn't get in touch. We expected never to find out what had happened to them.

Clearly, though, it was a friendship that wasn't meant to end so soon. When Sophie was a few months old, I was pushing her through Belsize Park in her pram. It was a beautiful, sunny, late-spring morning. Just outside our flat, I bumped into Harriet. She was out for her first walk with Finn who had been discharged from GOSH just a day or two before.

It was a special moment. We were so happy to see each other and felt so lucky to be out walking with our babies just like all the other local mums. I was overjoyed to learn that Finn had survived and was doing well. He still only weighed about five pounds. He looked tiny and incredibly fragile but he was there, he was alive … It felt like the final piece of a puzzle had fallen into place. We couldn't be one hundred per cent happy with the outcome of our story while we thought that Finn might have died. Our fates were somehow intertwined. For our story to have a completely happy ending, we needed theirs to as well.

After that chance meeting, Harriet and I started going for regular walks together. We filled each other in on the missing months in our stories and supported each other through the journey back to normality. Finn had spent four long and difficult months in NICU, during which he had faced many different life-threatening crises. Harriet and I understood each other and our experience of parenthood in a way that other parents with similar-age babies could not. We understood each other's worries and fears. We were still living with the knowledge that our babies might have developmental delays or learning disabilities. We had a different perspective to all of the other new parents we knew. They'd panic because their baby had a minor cold. Harriet and I were worried about lifelong disability.

Sophie and Finn still play together. As I watch them running around laughing, I can't help but picture them side by side in their incubators in the NICU. It seems only yesterday they were newborns lying in Room One fighting for their tiny lives. To think what they both went through to get here! They are a testament to the wonderful work of the NICU staff. Looking at them playing together it would never occur to you that they'd had such difficult infancies. They look like what they are – two carefree, happy, healthy four-year-olds having fun.

Nearly a year after Finn was born, Harriet and Danny finally got married at their original venue. Finn was a page boy. He was still very small and he was still very vulnerable, but he was there and he had a bright future ahead of him.

◊

There's a buzzer in the NICU. The emergency buzzer. It alerts the medics if there's an emergency and they need to come fast. It rings throughout the waiting room, the corridor and the nurseries. The staff can hear it wherever they are on the unit. Moments after it goes off, doctors and nurses fly out of nurseries and offices, down The Corridor to wherever they are needed to resuscitate a

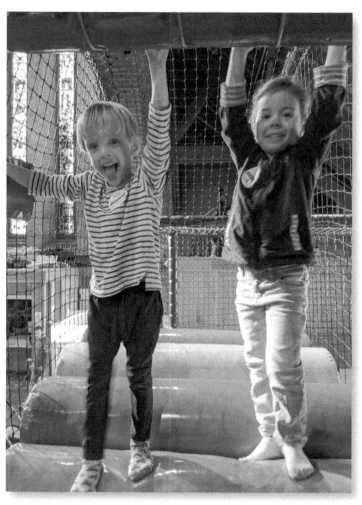

Sophie and Finn playing together at Finn's fourth birthday party

baby whose heart has stopped or to save a baby that has just been delivered on Labour Ward and is in trouble.

It's awful. It's one of the most stressful and upsetting parts of life on the unit. Each time the buzzer goes off, every parent who's not beside their baby turns pale and gets goosebumps. Hearts pound. Is it my baby? Why has the alarm been activated? Where are the doctors going? Is it in the direction of my nursery? No parent can breathe easily again until they have ascertained that the emergency didn't involve their baby. But if it didn't, that meant it was someone else's. And in some ways that's just as bad.

I don't think any parent gets used to that buzzer, however long they spend on the unit. It always spells possible catastrophe. I've heard plenty of parents who have spent time in NICU say they have flashbacks involving the buzzer. That when they hear a loud bell in normal life, it immediately takes them back to the stress of life in intensive care.

I'm hearing it for real in the afternoon, when the buzzer goes off as I walk back to Room One from The Dairy. It isn't for Sophie, but it could have been.

Just once during our time on the unit I witnessed the whole drama play out.

When Finn and Sophie were a few days old I was sitting beside Sophie. One of the senior consultants, Dr Angela Huertas-Ceballos, was in the room. Angela. I'd never met anyone so aptly named. She is the nearest thing to an angel: calm, kind, gentle and entirely capable. She exudes a Parisian glamour and speaks with a soft, South American lilt. Everyone who meets her seems to fall slightly in love with her. She'd be charming under any circumstances, but her position of power and her life-saving role on the unit added to her effect.

On this particular day, all was calm in Room One until, suddenly, the alarms on Finn's machines went crazy. Beep. Beep. Beep. Beep. I had become accustomed to the constant beeping of the kit in intensive care. I'd learnt to ignore most of the beeps. I'd even discovered the 'silence alarm' button on Sophie's monitor. This was different. These alarms meant business. They weren't going to be easily silenced. They were there to tell the staff something important. Very important.

Finn's heart had stopped. He had been taken off his ventilator to see if he could cope without it, which he had for a few hours. Then, suddenly and unexpectedly, he had crashed. He was dying. But he picked the right moment. Dr Huertas-Ceballos was there for him. She was beside him in an instant.

For a moment, I sat a few feet away and witnessed Dr Huertas-Ceballos saving Finn's life. The nurses were flapping around, pressing panic buttons and calling for back up, but Dr Huertas-Ceballos was dealing with it. Completely calm and unflappable. She didn't need back-up. She had it all under control. I watched in disbelief as she gave Finn CPR, using one finger to keep his miniscule heart pumping blood around his tiny, fragile body. He still weighed less than two pounds.

As Dr Huertas-Ceballos performed her delicate magic, she coolly instructed the nurses to intubate him again. To get him hooked back up to the ventilator. By the time back-up arrived, Dr Huertas-Ceballos had him safely back on the ventilator.

As soon as anyone had a moment, I was ushered out of the room along with the other parents present and, ominously, the blind over the window in the door of Room One was lowered. I found myself standing in The Corridor. My baby was behind the closed door and no one was allowed in. I was painfully aware of the significance of having been asked to leave the room, and of the blind having been closed. The nurses were protecting Finn's privacy. They didn't want strangers to witness his death.

But, thanks to Dr Huertas-Ceballos' life-saving intervention, he didn't die. They stabilised him again. Once they were confident that he was out of immediate danger, the blind was raised, the door opened and we were all allowed back in. Life returned to normal in Room One.

It was a terrifying reminder of how quickly disaster can strike in intensive care. How fragile the lives of these babies are. How fast everything can change for them – and their families. One minute, Finn was thought to be doing really well, coping without a ventilator for the first time. The next, his heart had stopped. The line between life and death in the NICU is perilously thin. In normal life, it feels as though there is a huge gulf between life and death. In the NICU it's a hair's breadth. The possibility of death hangs over you all the time.

◊

In the evening of this fourth day, Sophie is a little unstable. The doctors have to increase the amount of oxygen she is receiving, having been gradually reducing it. They think she has become stressed and agitated. Finn's arrival led to a period of busyness in the room and being able to wriggle around for the first time has worn her out.

She is so unwell that even little movements and brief periods of activity around her are more than she can cope with. To remain stable, she needs complete calm and immobility. The doctors insist that the blinds on the window beside her are kept closed and that she wears an eye mask and earplugs the whole time.

There are times when she is too unstable to have her nappy changed, even by the most experienced and gentle of neonatal intensive care nurses. However carefully and quickly they do it, it sends her vital signs haywire. Her oxygen saturation plummets. The situation is becoming normalised for us but, in reality, there is nothing normal about her situation. She is still on the very boundary between life and death. Everything could change in an instant.

February Thirteen

When we enter the room, we're confronted by a happy sight. Sophie is surrounded by fewer machines and the cap and EEG electrodes have been removed from her head. Gradually, she is escaping from some of the technology.

She has finished her three days of cooling and has returned to a normal temperature, which Jamie's diary records as thirty-six point six degrees. Much healthier than the thirty-three degrees she has been since the morning of her birth. The doctors are very relieved to see that she doesn't have any fits while she is being warmed up. We had been warned there was a risk that she might and that this would be a sign of brain damage.

As she has finished warming and her EEG results have been normal, this machine is removed. There is no longer a computer to the right of her cot showing a continuous trace of her brain activity. Nor does she any longer need the little white cap she's been wearing since she arrived at UCLH.

We can finally see all of her head! Her hair is full of little patches of glue where the electrodes have been attached. They agitate me. I want to look after my baby, to clean her up, to wash her hair, to remove the glue. But I can't.

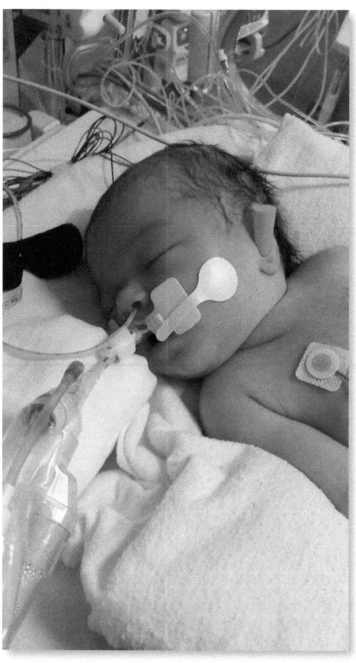

Sophie shortly after the EEG cap was removed – the glue that held the electrodes in place is still visible in her hair

As her mother, I am uncomfortable with having to leave her looking a mess. I want her to look cherished and well cared for. The nurses kindly offer to try to wipe the glue away but there's only a certain amount they can manage with cotton wool and water. They have to be careful not to overstimulate or distress her. Her stability is, after all, more important than her hairdo. Her hair still matters to me, though.

Despite a wobbly previous evening, the doctors have also been able to reduce her oxygen again. However, they have put her back on the muscle-paralysing medication because they feel that moving around stressed her. It feels like a step backward, seeing her fully sedated and paralysed again. But we understand and are happy with any intervention that the doctors feel will help to keep her stable.

◊

Jamie's diary

'Daddy has decided I should be kept abreast of what is happening in the world as I cannot go out and see it yet. So, he has started reading to me from The Week!

'Daddy got a bit low today because he was worried about me all day. So, Mummy sent him home to relax.'

◊

Jamie's way of coping with the situation, and with the helplessness of our position, is to try and understand everything that is going on. To empower himself as her father. He tries to learn the science, the medicine. To study all of Sophie's statistics, all of the details in her observations and all of her test results. They fluctuate throughout the day. Some of the time they're better than at other times. This is expected; it is normal for a baby in her situation. The doctors are relaxed about minor fluctuations, they understand what matters and what doesn't. They know what's behind the changes and whether the reasons are important or not.

But fixating on the numbers isn't really helping Jamie. It's just making him more stressed and upset. Every time she has a brief blip, he gets upset, watches the monitors constantly and obsesses over them. The nurses tell us to concentrate on the baby, not on the machines. I find that much easier than Jamie does, which is why I found this period easier than he did.

I'm happy to just look at Sophie and to trust what the doctors are telling me. And I strongly suspect that they are shielding us from some of the worst details. I think they tell us everything we need to know. That is, an honest description of her illness and her care, but they don't share unnecessarily upsetting details.

◊

I think I only realised it in retrospect but I think they got the balance right. We knew how ill she was. We didn't need to be scared any further. However, it meant that there are details I only learnt since she left hospital. For example, at some point during her time in intensive care Sophie developed aspiration pneumonia. I didn't know that at the time so it doesn't feature in this story. I don't know where it fits in. I only learnt that when Dr Huertas-Ceballos introduced a junior doctor on the unit to Sophie and her case, when she was one.

Jamie, on the other hand, needed to try and understand it himself. He would get Dr Kendall to give him detailed explanations of exactly what was wrong with Sophie and what the treatment aimed to achieve. He would insist on biology lessons. Fortunately, I think Dr Kendall was more than happy to deliver them and was probably delighted to have a parent who took so much interest in the medical details – in his art. He would appear in the room with little graphs he had made for Jamie to explain what was happening. This was extremely kind! He was always so busy and there was no need for him to do this. It certainly helped Jamie as much as any parent can be helped in this situation. And we will always be grateful for that.

◊

Back to Room One, with Sophie. To know how she's doing, witness any wobbles or fluctuations. We see the nurses caring for her and hear the doctors discussing her progress. We're in the loop.

When we leave the unit in the evening it's different. We have to assume that she remains as she was when we left. We know that if there are any significant changes, someone will call us. As a result, we begin to live in fear of our phones ringing. We are terrified of receiving a call in the middle of the night. We know that if our phones ring in the night, it will probably mean she has died.

Before we go to bed, we repeatedly check that they're on loud. That we're contactable.

When we're awake, if either of our phones ring, we immediately panic. Our hearts race until we look to see who's calling us. An unknown number causes spasms of panic. I remember being very sharp with a cold caller. Not because I really mind cold calls most of the time, but because it terrified me. I think I shouted at her to leave me alone; told her to think about what other people's lives might be like before bothering them unnecessarily. I informed her briskly I had a desperately sick baby in intensive care and needed to be available for the hospital to call. I think I even told the poor woman that when I had heard her call, I immediately assumed it meant my baby had died.

February Fourteen

Jamie

I religiously kept a diary while Sophie was in the NICU. It was a much-needed outlet for the emotions that we went through each day. I wrote it from Sophie's perspective and, as a result, kept very few details of what we were doing. Inevitably, the days all merged into one, and details have faded over time. However, I want to try and give a feel for what a 'typical' day for a NICU daddy is like.

◊

We wake up early from a deep sleep. After the stresses, emotions and adrenaline of the day we slip into a deep, dreamless sleep. We are lucky to have this important relief.

First, I feel a wave of relief as the rays of winter sunshine enter our bedroom window through the large tree outside our building. The long, vanilla blind is lazy about keeping us cocooned in darkness. We haven't had a phone call instructing us to go to the hospital. It would seem another eight hours have passed without our Sophie dying, or getting significantly closer to death. After the initial relief comes the desperate worry and fear. What news will we receive today?

We call the ward from our bedroom. We know the deal now. We know many of the nurses by name, though some remain forever nameless to us. Unknown strangers caring for our baby. We have to try several times to get through.

Yes. Sophie is okay. She was struggling a bit in the night. Her oxygen saturation dipped twice. They had to increase the oxygen levels and the frequency of the ventilator. She has had her feeds. She's doing a bit better now. The doctor will look at her infection markers later.

Dread. Stomach-churning fear. Desperation. Panicked hope. A feeling of helplessness. She's meant to be well. At the very least she should be getting better. She had a good day yesterday. Will she ever get better?

We get out of bed and prepare. All that matters in the world is our child in the hospital. Day-to-day tasks are done quietly, quickly and without much thought. Our minds and hearts are elsewhere. In that NICU cot. Toast. One slice. Butter not quite melted. Marmite. No appetite. Food is fuel so some bites are forced down but with no pleasure. I joke about the NICU diet being one of the most effective, even if it comes at a high price.

Emma is calm and practical. Around half-past-seven she summons a black cab on her app. Down the three flights of stairs from the top floor. Plush carpet. White walls. Victorian stucco of a townhouse villa converted for five families to live in. Our little home in our favourite part of London. Now it feels like a whole neighbourhood in dust sheets. Inaccessible to us because our own private world is upside down. All normal things made strangers because they're no longer what matters to us.

Into the black cab. It's sunny, clear and crisp. The cab driver is cheery. Emma makes small talk as she does so well. They probably get onto why we are going to hospital. The cabbie is sympathetic and positive in the stereotypical, East Londoner, salt of the earth way. Why do they never act like that with me? Perhaps I bring out the worst in them.

London road signs. London buses. More traffic. Fewer leaves. Nearly at the hospital. The big road junction near Euston, all ways blocked with traffic. A stressful and hectic space that acts like an echo chamber to my own fears. Even now, years later, my blood pressure rises when I go near.

'Just drop us off at the back.' There's a good spot for cabbies to pull in just next to the entrance.

The UCLH building is not bleak like many NHS hospital buildings. It's an imposing skyscraper with a white frame and large blue-tinted windows. It feels relatively cutting edge and modern. Leafy Bloomsbury is not far away, and the Oxbridge college-like buildings of the old UCL campus give a more secure feel to the back of the hospital where we are dropped off.

Dread, fear, hope. That knot of anxiety in the stomach. Slightly nauseous. The cabbie's paid automatically through the app. Little things like not faffing around with cash are a blissful relief. The banality of pointless or frustrating tasks makes them unbearable in this new context of ours. I can completely understand how people who have lost everything, or who are at risk of losing everything, can act in extraordinary ways. One's normal compass on everything from mortality to day-to-day human convention evaporates remarkably quickly.

The automatic doors slide open. Past the reception desk and the vending machines. Who can eat at a time like this? Into the lift. Emma is still sore from the birth. Stoic and slightly senseless, she's been cavorting about. I've been a bad husband and not forced her to slow down. The stitches holding her episiotomy together have torn and she's on antibiotics. She makes no fuss but is obviously very uncomfortable. We take the lift to spare her climbing the stairs to the second floor. For the eighth time, I read the notice about washing hands and the display about Elizabeth Garrett Anderson who the building is named after. Elizabeth will be Sophie's middle name.

The lift opens. Over to the NICU entrance. Ring the buzzer and wait. Hope a doctor or staff member comes by with a pass. Intercom clicks. 'We are here to see Sophie in Room One.' Door buzzes open. Hand sanitiser gel. That sharp, sweet, sickly scent. Drop off our day bag in the locker. Did we even pack it? When? Emma must have done it because she is sensible and is bringing in the breastmilk she has expressed.

The waiting room is the same as when, completely broken, I first entered it on the morning Sophie was admitted. Plastic waiting room chairs. The wall of lockers for parents. Some parents move in for months. A door to a frequently used WC. A consulting room. The matron's room. The reception office. The sinks beside the red line taped onto the floor. The taps have weird, long, one-way handles. There's strong soap and stronger hand sanitiser. The water comes out fast and scalding hot. The ritual begins. Scald, soap, scrub. Scald, soap, scrub. Paper towels. Apply hand sanitiser. You do this every time you cross a red line. Each time. Each line. There are at least two red lines before we reach Sophie. We brace ourselves. Reality will be staring us in the face soon. There's no more hiding from what we fear and treasure most.

Two left turns down the corridor. Past the lower dependency nurseries for babies who aren't as close to death as Sophie is. Each nursery has glass windows, but blinds are usually drawn to provide some privacy for the little souls ensconced in their incubators. Like four little islands in a medical sea, each surrounded by a small flotilla of parents and staff. We walk past the staff desk on the left where the senior nurses monitor vital signs from all the beds. They carry out the hundreds of tasks involved in keeping more than thirty babies alive who would have died had nature had been allowed to take its course. Today the desk is empty except for one senior nurse with glasses. We walk past her quickly to the last room on the corridor. Room One. For the sickest babies.

We walk across another red line. As we enter, we look toward the back-left corner where Sophie's cot is, hungry to learn what the current state of play is. There are nurses in the room but not around her bed. Usually a good sign. We turn to the sinks on the left, tucked into the corner. Scalding water. Soap. Scrub. Dry. Hand sanitiser.

Emma approaches Sophie directly. She says something motherly like 'hello my darling girl'. Strokes her head. I glance at Sophie's stats on the monitor above her bed. My whole emotional state is wrapped up in whether or not they look okay. The doctors have told me repeatedly to ignore these and focus on her instead. The numbers are for them to worry about. I can't possibly follow their advice.

Heart rate and blood pressure look okay. Oxygen saturation fluctuating between ninety-seven per cent and ninety-six per cent. Nothing disastrous. But only one hundred per cent ever really helped me to relax. Like even the slightest turbulence on an aeroplane, the smallest deviation from 'healthy' immediately switches on what I believe therapists would call my catastrophising tendency. Impending doom at any moment. The thing is that, now, these worst-case fantasies feel a lot more like reality. Planes do sometimes just plummet out of the sky.

There she is. On her side. She still wears the eye mask and ear plugs. She's sedated and her physical senses dulled to prevent excessive stimulation to her little brain. We're told to talk to her as it will comfort her. Seems like a bit of a contradiction in terms, but it gives us something to do. Her skin looks pinker today, though she's becoming bloated from water retention. She looks like a healthy, chubby baby but we know this water weight is becoming a problem. It's putting strain on her kidneys and, more importantly, it increases fluid in the lungs, making pneumonia more likely.

The oscillating ventilator is strapped to her mouth. The strange machine pulsates rhythmically. Kind of like a rapid pneumatic drill or mechanised tyre pump. Her torso vibrates as the pressure fluctuates in her ribcage. It is totally unnatural, but it has kept her alive these last few days and we're grateful for that.

Sophie's bed is by the window. This allows for some natural light and a view out to the medical buildings beyond. It's hardly scenic but it helps to make it feel a bit less claustrophobic and panic inducing. The sound of machines keeping babies alive and the pinging of monitors create a sense of foreboding at the best of times, and the occasional crisis at a cot immediately raises one's blood pressure. However, most the time it's relatively calm.

I stroke Sophie's head. Hold her little hand. Is there anything more perfect than a baby's hand? Perfection in miniature. Soft. I think our hands are underappreciated. I think they represent much about what it is to be human. What it means to be unique. What it means to care or create. The power to heal or kill. In a baby's hand there is no sin. Only good things yet to come. They clasp their little fingers around yours in an instinctive act of need. One of the first acts of love a parent will receive from their child.

The nurse comes over to the bed. Good. It's Marion today. One of the nurses we like best because she's clearly very competent and honest. Not one to sugar-

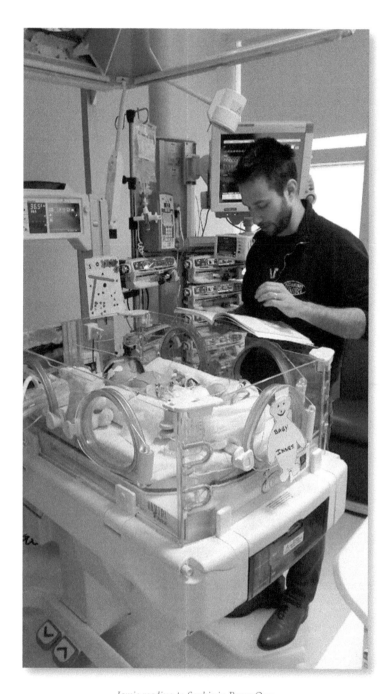

Jamie reading to Sophie in Room One

coat things so you can trust her and can be a little more positive when she says something good. She is a short, middle-aged woman. Strong German accent. Her face is kind and reassuring. She's says good morning and we make NICU small talk as she checks Sophie's multiple cables, empties the urine from the catheter bag, takes notes from her stats and marks them in her file at the end of the bed. She works quickly and with care, her movements efficient and well practised.

We still feel like we're holding glass when we get close to Sophie, so scared are we of accidentally unplugging a cable or wire. From our talk with Marion I always try to divine whether the picture is good or bad. Today it is mixed. It seems the key will be to wait for the infection marker test results to come back, then they will be discussed on the ward round. It is set at a fixed time but the doctors are always late as they make their pilgrimage from bed to bed.

Emma goes to what I call the milking parlour, a mothers-only room where chairs, sterilised bottles and breast pumps await. She'll fill several bottles of breastmilk which will be fed to Sophie via syringe and nasal tube. It's hardly romantic but the doctors are adamant that it's the best sustenance for Sophie. It also gives Emma a purpose and specific connection with Sophie. A little bit of normal in an abnormal world. As well as that, it's a den of motherly sisterhood, where the women get a chance to gossip about the medical staff, to rant about a less capable nurse, or to share their woes.

There isn't really an equivalent for the fathers. Unavoidably, the fathers on the unit are often a bit like lost souls. The mothers can be maternal, to an extent, but fathers cannot protect or provide. We are helpless and pointless. I don't have a single conversation with another father in the hospital. There isn't the context in which it would happen. I am also too stressed and upset to feel like striking up conversations with strangers.

While Emma pumps milk, I help Marion with the feed. Ten millilitres of milk in a tiny syringe. We hook it up to the tube in her nose. There is a specific set of steps to be followed to make sure it's done hygienically and safely. I've done it a few times now so I'm allowed to do it largely unaided. I push the syringe down very slowly.

Minutes pass before it's all gone. Her stomach is very small and if I do it too quickly, she will vomit it all back up, which only adds to the sense of foreboding. If I can only help her keep this feed down that is one more step to being okay, I think. She keeps this one down, thank God.

We have a little drawer of things for ourselves in the bedside table, just below the clever system of automatic syringes that pump about six different medicines at a steady rate into Sophie. They include a strong muscle relaxant, anti-inflammatories, and morphine for pain relief. We have a copy of *The BFG* so I stand by her bed and read it to her. I have not read it since she left intensive care. Too many associations. I'm not sure about the purpose of reading *The BFG* to Sophie but it gives me something to do. Moments of clarity bubble up as I read and I shed a tear quietly onto the pages.

Emotions are always running high. Emma returns from the milking parlour, and takes over being mother hen. I sit for a bit and look around. Some specialists have been monitoring another baby in another bed. She's hooked up to the same device to measure brain activity as Sophie was. Brain damage is still a concern with Sophie, but so far they are happy that she seems to have dodged anything too serious. There's still hope she may be okay. The parents of this baby are a little more reserved. I watch the facial expressions of the doctors as they scrutinise the results. I can't help but overhear their quiet conversation. I may be misinterpreting the situation but it seems like an unhappy case.

The baby is relatively well overall – certainly healthier than Sophie. But readings of the brain activity on the screen look very different to Sophie's. I very carefully interrogated the technician who carried out Sophie's EEG, asking what he looks for in the readings. He told me about the general background hubbub of electrical signals which are what constitute consciousness in all of us; about the healthy variations in activity between sleep cycles, and how these sleep cycles evolve in young babies. He told me about the tell-tale signs of seizures and epileptic fits, with the sudden spikes in the wrong kinds of activity. I don't think it looks promising for the baby in the opposite corner to Sophie. I never learnt what happened to her.

As a species, humans adapt quickly to changes in circumstances and judge our relative state compared to others in the same environment. Sophie is one of the sickest babies in London, and yet we now judge her condition comparative to those around us. Is it bad that

I take some selfish relief from the fact that at least Sophie is not having fits like the child on the other side of the room; that if she survives, she won't be as severely brain damaged?

The doctors finally arrive for their ward round. Serene and glamorous Dr Huertas-Ceballos. Dr Kendall with his earnest energy and shed-sized brain concealed behind a bespectacled face. They look at the notes and ask the nurses questions. We, in turn, ask questions. The answers are often the same. She's very sick. When she gets better, she will get better fast. She should do. Issues around secondary infections and inflammation markers. A new course of antibiotics. Adjustments to nitrogen, oxygen and machine frequency. A mixture of dread and optimism.

Soon after they leave the physio arrives. The process is brutal to watch – a bit like a rugby player contorting a toy bear. I flee to the family room as I find it unbearable to watch. The small cramped space doesn't bring much solace. It's always full of shocked or stressed parents. It often stinks of the hospital food that can be ordered by new arrivals or those who can't bring themselves to leave the building.

I sit down to read the same posters on the walls and make a cup of tea. The emergency alarm goes off. Parents' eyes racing each other to see the bed number. Thank God it is not mine! Once I was there when it was the child of a mother in the room. She left with a lurch and a sob. It wasn't the first time it had been her turn.

I message Emma to say I'm going for lunch. Does she want anything? She'll get something later. I leave the building feeling sick and not at all hungry and make my way across to the UCL student union café. It's both a blissful relief to be somewhere else and an overwhelmingly forceful reminder that this is no longer my world. It's a world full of young, hopefully carefree people, on their laptops, drinking their flat whites. Our world is small and fearful now. Sandwich, crisps, drink. Some of it gets eaten. None with any pleasure. Heading back inside, one foot wishes to hurry to check all is well. The other wants to run away.

I give Emma a hug after going through the handwashing ritual, then send her off to get some food too. She's still recovering from her own ordeal. What a darling she is! I stare at Sophie's face, hold her hand, and talk to her about the bedroom waiting for her at home, her grandparents, games we will play when she is older and better. Once again, I feel this is more for me than her. Medical care in the NICU is part child physiology, part parental sanity.

The hours pass. The staff come and go. Sophie's vital stats go up and down. At one stage the machine starts bleeping. Her oxygen saturation has fallen below ninety percent. The nurse hurries over, mutes the machine, and changes some settings on another machine. Things stabilise over the next thirty minutes. By the end of our stay, I will be confidently muting the alarms on the machine, aware of what does and does not matter. I could have had a decent go at adjusting the medical equipment, but obviously I never did. Time passes slowly, with a great pressure on our heads. Like a millstone slowly grinding over us. Tomorrow Granny and Grandpa will be coming to visit, and Natalie is due in the afternoon. That will be nice.

The shifts change early in the evening. Another day has almost passed. Sophie's alive but no better. Each step forward is followed by another step backward. We are exhausted yet have contributed nothing. We start to get our things together. Talk to the evening shift doctors about her progress. Look to see which nurses will be looking after her overnight. We kiss our darling little baby goodnight but cannot take her with us. So small and so poorly. So precious. Leaving is simultaneously a wrench of loss as we surrender all parental instincts to a room of strangers, while also a blessed relief to be away from the immediate source of our sickening worry, and a place where we are hounded by alarms and beeps and buzzers and bright lights. Away from words like pulmonary hypertension, secondary infection, pneumonia, oxygen saturation and auto-injectors.

Exhausted, we sit in the black cab that takes us back up the hill. We hold hands across the backseat. Too tired to talk. Into our small flat. Homely and safe, but into it we take our fear like an infection. We shower to rid ourselves of the hospital smell and London detritus. We make a meal which neither of us eat properly. No alcohol because we may be called to the hospital at any time. Then some trashy TV which we don't take in. We make conversation but can't remember what we've said. Before bed we call the ward to check in. She's doing okay. No real change. Sleep comes quickly, but our thoughts are with Sophie, and our last thought is:

'Please let the phone not ring in the night'. Then our brains reset to zero, ready to do it all again tomorrow.

◊

I wrote in my diary:

> 'Daddy woke me up this morning by singing me a silly song about drunken sailors. Apparently, you need to put them in a long boat with a hosepipe on them … Useful advice!'
> …
> 'Overall, Daddy tells me that I'm doing well. I'm not ready for cuddles quite yet but I'm definitely a bit more stable and taking baby steps in the right direction.
> 'I asked Daddy what he was looking forward to most and he said:
> 1. Cuddling me close
> 2. Kissing me on my little head
> 3. Seeing me snuggle with my Mummy.
> …
> 'Today Dr Kendall was very positive about my progress. I've been stable and well behaved all day … so far!'

◊

Emma

Sophie is having another good day. Her infection markers are dropping and the doctors are proceeding with their efforts to wean her off some of her drugs and support.

143

Although Sophie has had a good day, I am struggling. I had multiple stitches after my episiotomy. I should be slumped on a sofa at home cuddling my baby and healing. Instead, I'm marching up and down the four flights of stairs to our flat, navigating the Northern Line and its many stairs and escalators, traversing hospital corridors and have nothing but an uncomfortable stool to sit on all day.

My episiotomy wound is painful and I have no access to painkillers in the NICU. When I can bear the pain no longer I ask Jamie's sister, Natalie, to go to the Boots outside the hospital to grab me some. Why I thought I could cope without painkillers immediately after giving birth, I have no idea. Bravado, I suppose. Clearly, I should have furnished myself with some.

The episiotomy wound is also bleeding heavily every time I go to the bathroom. And I'm still bleeding profusely from the birth. Every time I walk up the stairs, unload the washing machine or carry bags of shopping I start to bleed even more heavily.

My body is sending a clear message that I'm overdoing it. I'm going to have to stop thinking solely of Sophie and start looking after myself. This irritates me. I should respect my body and be understanding toward it. It's been through a huge ordeal. But I'm not. I'm frustrated that it's letting me down. I think it should stop making a fuss and let me concentrate on my baby.

My parents give me a cheque and strict instructions to stop taking the tube to and from the hospital and to start getting taxis instead. More urgently, though, I have to get my stitches seen to. Going to the loo has become intensely stressful because any straining causes blood to start dripping from the wound. I'm too scared to look at it and I have no idea what is going on down there. I just don't have the emotional energy for it. Worrying about Sophie is all I can manage. The fact my own body is also suffering is more than I can bear. I have to try and get it sorted out, for everyone's sake.

So, rather than going straight to see Sophie in the morning, I go back to the Maternity Department at our local hospital and ask them to look at my stitches for me. It's exasperating that I spend my whole time at UCLH but have to go to a different hospital to have my own medical needs attended to. It seems entirely illogical. It's time-consuming and inconvenient. Most importantly, it keeps me away from Sophie.

At the local hospital it's chaotic. They're very busy. They have more urgent cases to attend to. I have to wait for a long time. Eventually, I am seen and the harassed midwife agrees to check on the stitches.

She takes one look, tuts to herself and says: 'Yes. All of your stitches have come undone. You have a gaping wound there now.'

She then proceeds to draw a diagram of it on my notes. I still have it in a drawer of our desk. A quick biro sketch of my nether regions with a large tear in them.

I ask what is to be done about it.

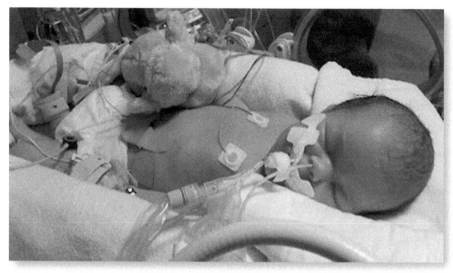

*Sophie in NICU on February 14. Her head is visibly
swollen because of severe fluid retention*

Emma with Sophie on February 14, 2016, in NICU

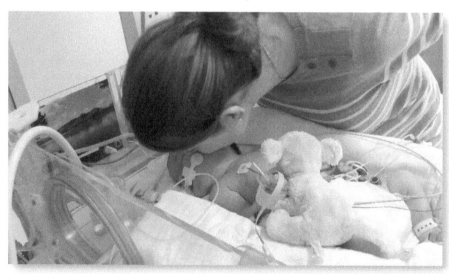

She says: 'Nothing.' She tells me their policy isn't to re-stitch stitches that have come undone but just to leave them to heal on their own. She says it will just mean that they will take longer to heal. She also gives me preventative antibiotics to ensure the wound doesn't become infected.

It's helpful to know what the problem is but it's also upsetting. Before this, I had proceeded on the basis that I was recovering well. Now I know that I'm walking around with a 'gaping wound' that is bleeding heavily and may take weeks to heal. It makes me feel vulnerable and defenceless. I'm also very reluctant to take the antibiotics. I really don't like taking medication. I'm worried they will come with side effects that will make my life even more difficult. I don't think I could cope with antibiotic-induced nausea all day on the unit.

It is, however, a useful wake up call. I will now make more effort to be careful with myself, and Jamie has started policing my activity levels closely, telling me off every time I take the stairs rather than the lift in the hospital, or empty the dishwasher rather than asking him to do it for me.

◊

This was not the only time that our health caused us anxiety while Sophie was in NICU. Everyone on the unit is acutely aware that the babies, particularly the very premature ones, are terribly vulnerable to infections. As a result, there is an unwritten rule – a code of conduct – that no one enters the unit if they are even slightly under the weather. What might be a mild cold for a healthy adult, could be catastrophic for an extremely preterm baby with an underdeveloped immune system.

We were very conscious of this from Sophie's perspective. It was February; there were lots of bugs going around. The last thing she needed was to catch 'flu from us. We were also very aware of it from the perspective of other babies. We were terrified by the thought that we could carry a bug onto the unit that could harm someone else's baby.

As a result, we became hyperaware of our own health. A slight cough that we would normally barely have registered suddenly becomes a cause for panic. It is twofold: we are terrified of passing something on to the babies; we also dread not being able to go to the unit to be with Sophie. The thought of getting a bad cold and not being able to see her for days at a time is horrendous.

We are both feeling ropey because of the circumstances – we are sleep deprived, stressed and emotionally drained and are spending our entire time in a hospital room. Not to mention the fact that I've just given birth. But the tiredness, aches and pains, and general lack of wellbeing take on a whole new meaning. We start to analyse our symptoms and to discuss whether they are a reason for staying away from the unit. We desperately want them not to be, but we also want to be sure we are safe to go in. The priority has to be Sophie's health, not our desire to be with her.

It is a difficult balance. We have to accept that it is inevitable that we aren't going to be feeling our best at this time but we need to work out whether we have anything contagious. The more we think about it, the worse we feel. Real symptoms became mingled with psychosomatic ones. Anxiety begins to create its own symptoms.

Thankfully, neither of us developed any symptoms concerning enough to force us to stay away. That would have been torturous. We'd have felt so guilty not being with her while she was fighting for her life. We would have felt like negligent parents not being there for her and not being present to hear the doctors' updates. We would never have been able to relax and to rest at home. Every ounce of us was being drawn to the unit and to our baby.

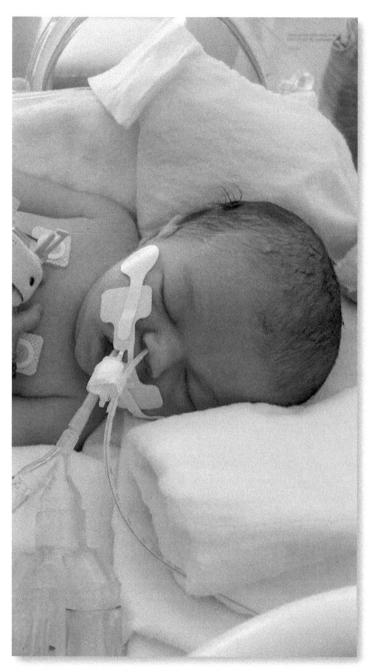

Sophie in NICU at six days old

February Fifteen

Sophie is now almost a week old. Initially, the doctors had told us that she would be extremely unwell for about a week but then she should turn a corner and start to improve very rapidly. Everyone's now waiting anxiously for this sudden improvement. We've reached the point at which it should happen. But it hasn't. And there isn't really any sign of it.

Within the next couple of days, she really needs to start getting much better. If she doesn't, her eventual recovery will be in doubt. She needs to demonstrate that she will eventually be able to cope without a ventilator. It's becoming very stressful. Until this point, we knew she was expected to be very sick, that she was following the expected path, so we could accept her situation and still hope that things would get better. Now, she is no longer meant to be like this. To know she is doing less well than her initial prognosis makes it even harder to bear.

Jamie's diary

'I am making some progress as the doctors have reduced the amount of nitric oxide I'm on. Hopefully I will come off this completely later today.

'However, this morning my lungs were not so good so they had to turn up the ventilator and oxygen.'

This is precisely what's not supposed to be happening. She's supposed to be needing less support. Not more. Dr Kendall is continuing to be cautiously optimistic but we can see that he's becoming slightly concerned. He's thrown everything he has at her – skill, knowledge, drugs and equipment. There's nothing more he could have done and she's supposed to have responded and started getting better. But she hasn't. She's still alive but she isn't much better than she was on the day she was born.

◊

Jamie's diary

'It's a lovely sunny day today and Daddy is reading still from *The BFG*. We're up to Chapter Eleven!

'I look super pretty today so Daddy's been taking lots of photos of me.'

◊

We have a lot of photos of Sophie's time in hospital. Initially, I didn't take many. It seemed inappropriate somehow. Like an invasion of her privacy. People take photos of happy moments they want to remember. Why would I want pictures of her on life support?

However, Dad encouraged me to take some. He told me that one day Sophie would be interested to see them. He painted a picture of us spending an evening in front of the fire, as a family, with a sixteen-year-old Sophie who would be interested to see what her first few weeks looked like. I don't think I had, until that point, dared to imagine her as anything other than a tiny baby. The concept of her as a teenager was completely alien to me. But Dad was right. As soon as he said it, I knew he was right. I knew it was important to have a record of this time because, for better or for worse, it was part of her story and, therefore, part of ours. She deserved the chance to know about it, if she survived, and if she wanted to.

◊

Having been on the unit for nearly a week, I'm now familiar with The Dairy and its idiosyncrasies. I'm also effortlessly producing numerous bottles of milk a day. Far more than Sophie can take. The NICU freezer is rapidly filling up with them. So much so that my milk supply has become near-legendary on the unit. Mums struggling to produce a few millilitres look on enviously. And I receive much praise from the nurses looking after Sophie for providing them with so much sustenance for her.

Being naturally skinny, I didn't think I looked like a likely source of plentiful milk. It surprises me that I am. But, while also feeling slightly like a dairy cow, I'm proud of the achievement. Providing lots of nourishment for Sophie feels like the one tangible thing I can really do for her. It means the nurses never need to worry about what to give her for her next feed.

◊

Once Sophie was able to breastfeed, this actually became problematic. She hadn't got the chance to practise with tiny quantities of colostrum. I produced so much milk that it practically drowned her every time she tried to master the art of feeding. She'd end up coughing and spluttering under the deluge. She eventually worked out a technique for getting the milk she wanted but no more. Unfortunately for me, this technique involved allowing all of the excess milk to pour out of the side of her mouth as she fed.

Initially, I found myself having to change both of our clothes every time I fed her because we were both soaked in milk. Then my ancient grandmother said, 'It is quite simple. Tuck a nappy into your bra every time you feed her – it will absorb the excess milk and keep you both clean.'

For want of a better idea I thought I'd give it a go. I assumed it would be a short-term solution while she learnt to take more milk in one go. Granny's strategy worked. It was great and saved me a huge amount of laundry. However, Sophie never did learn to feed without making a horrendous mess. So for a year I always fed her with a nappy tucked into my bra. The financial and environmental impact doesn't bear thinking about. It did, however, make breastfeeding her more practical.

To this day I wonder why she never learnt to feed properly. Was it just because she didn't get a chance to practise when she was tiny? Or was there more to it?

Our son, George, never spilled a drop of milk during the year that I fed him. Why did Sophie? I had a nagging worry that it was a sign of some tiny form of brain damage, even though, thinking about it now, that seems improbable.

◊

The Dairy itself is extremely odd. There sit a row of women, with their tops yanked up, attached to electric breast pumps. Just like dairy cows on a farm. It's an inevitable comparison to draw. It's essentially the same. But it isn't a thought I feel entirely comfortable with. I get used to the process to an extent, but my role as dairy cow never sits comfortably. There's something very industrial about it. Using the breast pumps completely removes all of the tenderness, intimacy and love that goes with breastfeeding a baby. It achieves the same end of nourishing the baby but in a horribly sanitised way.

Mums new to The Dairy always sit in awkward silence, concentrating on trying to produce their milk and get out of there as quickly as possible. Those who have been on the unit longer have become relaxed about the process. We are, after all, in there multiple times every day. These mums are relaxed about being half-naked in front of strangers. They are also so well practised at expressing milk that they don't have to think about it.

These mums sit there chatting on the phone. You aren't allowed to use your phone in the nurseries so it's useful dead time for catching up with people. Or, they gossip with the other mums. In this room, I learn which nurses don't get on, which doctors the nurses like and which

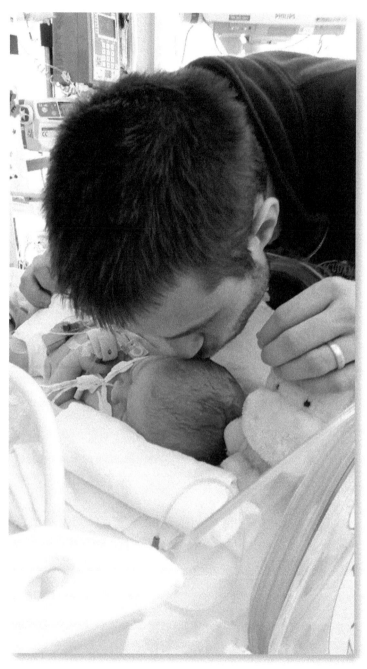

Jamie with Sophie on February 15, 2016

they are scared of, which parents are difficult to deal with and which are in the most difficult situations. For example, I hear about one poor lady who has extremely premature twins, one of whom is at GOSH, the other at UCLH, so she is having to split her time between the two hospitals. After months in intensive care, one son survives, tragically the other doesn't.

Conversations in The Dairy can be difficult. Some days everyone I meet there is just having a standard day and so it's straightforward. Other days, the atmosphere is much more emotionally charged. One mum might be elated because she is expressing in hospital for the last time before her baby is discharged, while another's baby has just deteriorated significantly. You always have to tread carefully with the questions you ask and the topics of conversation you choose. No one wants to inadvertently add to another mother's anguish.

February Sixteen

We're on our eighth day as parents and walk into Room One desperately hoping to hear good news. Hoping Sophie will have had a good night and will have started to show signs of the expected improvement. She should be needing less support. Maybe the doctors will have been able to reduce the amount of oxygen she's receiving? Maybe she no longer needs the nitric oxide? Possibly she'll soon be taken off the oscillating ventilator. Could she now cope on a normal ventilator?

Quite the opposite is the case. She's deteriorated significantly overnight and is back on the maximum support the unit can offer. The mood has changed. Faces are serious and it feels like hope is fading. She is, once again, as sick as a baby can be and still be alive. The doctors are now obviously really worried.

Dr Huertas-Ceballos provides a reassuring presence. She explains that she's awaiting test results but that she suspects Sophie has developed another serious infection. And that she has serious fluid retention because she isn't moving enough to shift the fluid around her body and that this is putting further pressure on her already struggling lungs.

As ever, even in the face of catastrophe, Dr Huertas-Ceballos is completely calm and collected. Crucially, she also has a plan. She puts Sophie on a new course of antibiotics in a bid to treat the suspected infection. She also slashes the amount of fluid she is being given to try and reduce the retention and, therefore, the pressure on her lungs.

This really is Sophie's last chance. If Dr Huertas-Ceballos' educated guess is wrong, if the treatment she suspects is needed isn't right, she will die. Soon. Dr Huertas-Ceballos is having to work on experience and gut feeling. She can't wait for test results to make clear what's going on in Sophie's tiny body. For a conclusive diagnosis. There isn't time. She would die before the results came back. She needs emergency treatment now.

The doctors optimistically explain what they think is wrong with Sophie and what they are doing about it. We don't know enough about neonatal medicine to understand just how bad things are.

◊

Years later, Natalie told me that on that day the extremely experienced neonatal intensive care nurse looking after Sophie admitted that she didn't think Sophie would survive the night.

This nurse had been looking after her all week. She had got to know Sophie and her illness. She had been hopeful about her until this point. Clearly, she now felt that hope was lost. She had fought for this baby for twelve hours a day and now believed that her efforts had been in vain.

159

She thought she would hand over to the nightshift a baby who would die on them. She thought she would come in the following morning, not to spend another day looking after Sophie, but to be told she was 'gone'.

While I didn't know at the time that the nurse had said this, I also felt hope was fading. That evening I emailed my godmother:

> 'Sophie has had a bad twenty-four hours. She's deteriorated a lot and is back on maximum support. She will now need to overcome this new infection and the fluid retention before she can return to trying to recover from her original problems.
> 'It is a complete roller coaster. I think the last twenty-four hours have been the hardest yet.'

I can still hear my own exhaustion and despair in this email. Usually, I'd write my godmother a long, chatty, jolly email. Clearly on that day I had neither the energy nor the spirit left to do so. I told her what she needed to know but with no embellishment. I'm sure the tone of it will have told her everything about both Sophie's situation and my emotional state.

In fact, later, when we looked at this email together, and her response, she admitted that while her reply was heartfelt, she had no real idea of the ordeal being endured. That it wasn't until she read this book that she fully understood.

She said: 'I confessed that, however appalling the possible tragedy, there was something about you, your stoicism or stiff upper lip, that made it hard to communicate on the level of depth the crisis so clearly called for.

'While I tried to offer help, it was as though somehow you couldn't absorb that help at the time. I fear that I didn't fully pick up on the tone of that email. I naturally mirrored your matter-of-fact manner in my reply. I wish, now, that I had better read your state and offered greater comfort.'

This conversation, which was only had as part of the editing of this book, was interesting but it was also a little upsetting. As I wrote above, I'd assumed that my godmother had understood and appreciated the suffering we were enduring. She and I are very close and usually, to use a cliché, she can read me like a book. I can now see that the danger of the stiff upper lip is that it hides suffering in a way that makes others believe support or comfort is not necessary.

In retrospect, I think I was probably a victim of my own stoicism throughout the experience. It resulted in others looking to me for comfort. At the time I was fine with that, I was coping and I was able to offer emotional support to Jamie in particular, when he was struggling. I suspect, though, that I would have been better off showing my own vulnerability and accepting more help.

◊

That night, I lie in bed thinking about planning Sophie's funeral. I fret that I don't even know how to go about planning a funeral. That I've no idea how we would want it to be. What music or readings we might want.

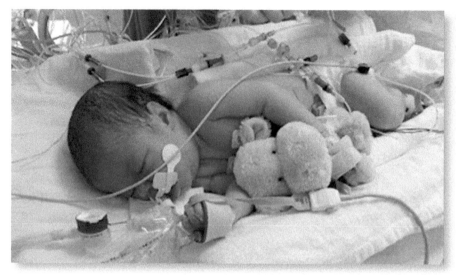

Sophie swollen with fluid retention

*This is the only photo we have of Sophie from February 16. Emma
took this one because it was the first time we had seen her face
free of a ventilator, feeding tube etc. They were only removed
very briefly while another procedure was being carried out*

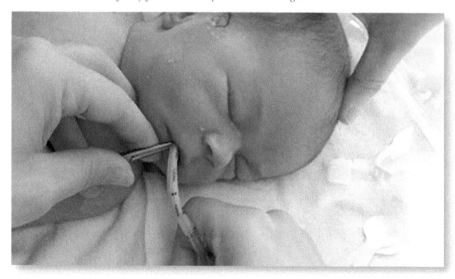

I lie there wondering how I can possibly be planning a funeral in the same week that I have become a mother, learnt that my new baby was desperately ill, sat beside her willing her to live and faced her imminent death.

It would be odd to invite family and friends to the funeral of a baby they have never met. It's only me and Jamie, my parents and Jamie's mum and sister who have met her. Why would people attend a funeral for someone they don't know? Someone who has never had the opportunity to enter their lives. I decide it would just have to be a very small affair for immediate family.

I wonder what to do with all the baby things we got for Sophie in preparation for her arrival and which remain untouched in our flat. Would we keep them safe for another baby or are they too inextricably linked to her? Would we think they are bad luck? Would we feel comfortable putting a new baby, a different baby, in his or her dead older sister's clothes? I imagine living in a flat full of Sophie's things once Sophie has gone and the thought is unbearable. I want them gone. Even now, while she is still alive, I wish none of the things were here. They are staring at me as a reminder that the baby who should be using them is dying. I don't want to have to look at them anymore.

◊

But hang on! I think I missed something from my account of the day. So much had happened it's hard to remember the chronology of events. Perhaps this wasn't such a bad day. I think this was the day, just as we reached the depths of despair, that another of the angels who looked after Sophie appeared on the scene.

Natalie had made contact with a friend of hers to say that her niece was receiving cooling on the NICU at UCLH. This friend's uncle, Professor John Wyatt, just happened to have been the doctor who pioneered the use of cooling for newborns. He had been in charge of the UCLH NICU for years but was now retired. He got in touch with Jamie to offer his support and he sent his regards to Dr Huertas-Ceballos, who had been one of his students.

Having been in touch by email, he called Jamie while we were in the hospital. Jamie left Room One to talk to him and they had a long conversation. Jamie explained the desperation of Sophie's situation and Professor Wyatt detailed the medical side of her illness and offered Jamie reassurance. Generously, he also said he would come to the unit to assess her if that would help. Jamie was so grateful for his warmth and for the comfort he offered.

When we mentioned the call to Dr Huertas-Ceballos, she was unreserved in her praise for him. As I recollect it, she described him as 'the God of neonatal medicine'. She asked us to tell him that he was welcome back on the unit any time he liked.

Then, lo and behold, just as Sophie hit rock bottom, he appeared. Came to see if he could help. The consultants welcomed him with open arms and he joined them on their ward round. I remember the jokes about the ward round taking twice as long as usual as he shared pearls of wisdom about the treatment of all of the babies on the unit.

Then he got to Sophie. He spent a long time reviewing her history. He agreed that Dr Huertas-Ceballos had been right to put her on the new antibiotics and to reduce her fluids. However, he also suggested that she should reduce the amount of muscle paralysing medication. He felt that if she were able to move around a little bit, she would shift more of the fluid that was squashing her lungs. I remember the other doctors looking slightly concerned by this suggestion. They were clearly worried that moving might stress and destabilise her again; that she was too sick to cope with the stimulation of mobility. However, they trusted him and agreed to give it a go.

That was all we saw of him. He was on the unit for the morning then he disappeared. For the rest of the day, other parents came over asking who the amazing doctor we had brought in was. Saying that he had made helpful suggestions for their babies too.

I wrote to Mum:

> 'Sophie couldn't have been reviewed by a more knowledgeable or well-respected doctor.
> 'He said he's seen lots of babies like her and that, despite everything, he'd be "highly optimistic" about her. Those were his very words! Isn't that amazing?'

Maybe all hope wasn't lost, after all.

February Seventeen

When Sophie was first admitted to the NICU the doctors told us that she'd be extremely sick for roughly a week and then she'd turn a corner and suddenly improve very rapidly. They were right. Just a matter of hours earlier, we thought Sophie was going to die. Now, things have changed completely. She has reached the corner and is turning it very fast.

Overnight the doctors took her off the muscle paralysing medication on the advice of Professor Wyatt. This helped to shift the fluid that had built up as a result of her immobility. The antibiotics have also kicked in and her infection markers are falling.

◊

Sarah comes to give Sophie her daily physiotherapy. While she is working on her, she takes her briefly off the oscillating ventilator so she can move her around, and she uses a bag-valve mask to ventilate her instead. This creates a normal breathing action, unlike the oscillating ventilator. Suddenly, Sarah notices that now, when she moves Sophie over to the manual ventilator her vital statistics are better than they are on the oscillator. She suggests to the doctors that she might benefit from being moved off the oscillator and on to a conventional ventilator. The doctors agree to give it a go and she immediately responds well, meaning she requires less oxygen than before. And, for the first time in her life, she has a normal breathing action. Sarah observation is a major turning point for Sophie.

◊

Sarah gave Sophie physio every day while she was in intensive care. It was clearly extremely beneficial, but it was hard to watch because it was surprisingly brutal. It involved powerful manipulation of her fragile body. Jamie remembers it more clearly than I do and says he found it so distressing that he couldn't remain in the room.

Maybe, for the purpose of self-preservation, my mind has filtered out its brutality. The main thing I remember is that when Sarah finished the session, she'd reposition Sophie in her incubator using Blue Cow to support her body in the chosen position. I remember her always leaving Sophie looking as though she was cuddling him. That was sweet.

◊

Jamie's diary

'As the doctors took me off the muscle relaxant overnight, I've started to wriggle around now. I also opened my eyes and got to see Mummy and Daddy properly for the first time.

'Apparently, I have beautiful eyes and we all think they might be blue. Daddy says I'm very beautiful!

167

'Grandpa came to see me today. He is very sweet as he reads to me from *The BFG* and has begun teaching me my first words: 'Come on Charlton!'.

'The doctors said the probable cause of my relapse was an umbilical infection and too much water, but I'm hopefully making progress on both fronts now.'

◊

In intensive care machines beep constantly. They beep because a shunt has run out of the medication it's delivering, or because a baby's heart rate has dropped or because a patient's breathing rate is concerning. Most beeps don't really matter. Some do. We are learning which ones to ignore and which ones to take note of. When we first arrived on the unit, we panicked about every beep! We soon learnt which ones the nurses were completely relaxed about and we have become relaxed about them too.

I've now got to a stage where I barely notice the beeps while I'm in Room One. They've become white noise which my brain filters out. At least, I thought that had happened. I'm not conscious of being fussed by them while I'm with Sophie. However, after only eight days on the NICU, I have started to notice that now I'm travelling to the hospital by tube again, I jump at the sound of doors beeping as they open, and of ticket barriers beeping as they let me through, even at the microwave beeping to alert me it has finished. Beeps in everyday life have taken on a new, and unwelcome, importance. They agitate me.

February Eighteen

Even though Dr Kendall told us this would happen, it's unbelievable how quickly Sophie has suddenly improved. How she's gone from the brink of death, to there being talk of her leaving intensive care within two days. Forty-eight hours ago, I was thinking about her funeral. Now, she has had such a good night that we are having incomparable conversations. It's hard for us to comprehend how quickly her situation has changed. I expected any improvement to be very gradual, but it isn't.

Dr Kendall is now expecting to be able to wake her up, and take her off her ventilator, imminently, but first he needs to fit in some last-minute tests.

Sophie is transferred to an MRI-compatible incubator and we follow as she is wheeled out of the NICU, along endless corridors, into the main part of the hospital, and through the doors of the Imaging Department. We wait at the door as she's taken toward a space age machine for her MRI brain scan. It's like a big, white plastic doughnut emitting blue lights. We're told the MRI will take a while so we stroll back to NICU to await her return.

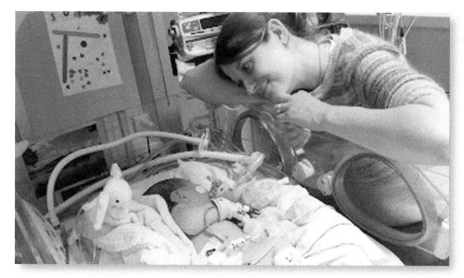

Emma with Sophie in the UCLH NICU on February 17

Sophie opening her eyes properly for the first time, February 17, 2016

Sophie on the morning of February 18, 2016, just hours before she was taken off her ventilator and was able to breathe for herself for the first time

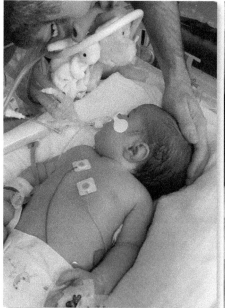

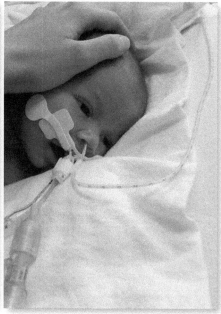

Once she's back, the doctors casually mention that she needs a lumbar puncture to check she doesn't have meningitis. In ordinary circumstances, parents would panic at the mere suggestion that their child might have meningitis. We just shrug and go along with it. We're used to near disaster, by this point. It's the norm.

We're asked to leave the room for this procedure. The staff let the parents remain next to their baby almost the whole time. I feel guilty leaving her but, as she is still sedated, she won't feel it and, overall, I'm glad I don't witness whatever happens behind those closed doors.

With the MRI and lumbar puncture complete, and her dependency on the ventilator hugely reduced, Dr Kendall begins to discuss waking her up and taking her off the ventilator altogether. To see how she copes without it. And, he's talking about doing it immediately!

Around lunchtime, she's gradually woken and her ventilator replaced with high-flow nasal oxygen therapy. She's now breathing for herself with just a little prong going into each nostril pushing extra oxygen into her lungs. Everyone is watching anxiously to see how she copes, breathing for herself for the first time in her life.

And she does it brilliantly!

Her oxygen saturation remains excellent and all her vital signs are stable. It's an enormous step forward. One that two days ago seemed an impossibility.

I'm astonished by her. Her strength and resilience. She's still so young and small and vulnerable-looking, but she has overcome so much. She's proved herself to be a true fighter. Jamie describes her as 'our little soldier'. I'm so proud of her that, after everything, she's now casually breathing for herself as though nothing has happened.

Dr Kendall reappears in the afternoon. He says he's delighted with how Sophie's doing. He explains that she will remain in intensive care overnight while they make sure she continues to cope without the ventilator. Then, if she's stable overnight, she will be moved to high dependency in the morning.

We are finally moving along The Corridor.

Critically, Dr Kendall also tells us that he has the preliminary results from Sophie's MRI. He says the scan showed a clinically insignificant bleed but that, otherwise, the results are completely normal. Ever reassuring and positive, he also explains that he suspects most babies who have recently been through the trauma of natural delivery probably have minor bleeds on their brains. It's just that most babies aren't given brain MRIs.

This is huge; some of the most important information we've been given since Sophie was born. Dr Kendall is not only giving Sophie a future; he's telling us he believes that future has every chance of being completely healthy. Despite the oxygen deprivation, despite the HIE, Dr Kendall doubts that Sophie has clinically significant brain damage. And we trust his every word.

Then, as if he hasn't already imparted enough joyous news, he casually adds that we can now hold Sophie for the first time. She's no longer on the ventilator, she's stable, so there's no reason why we can't hold her as soon as we're ready. We have been desperate for this moment. Now it's here it's almost overwhelming.

The nurse looking after her asks us if we would like to hold her straight away. Jamie kindly suggests that I should be the first to hold her. I sit awkwardly in a hospital armchair next to her incubator and watch as slowly, carefully, the nurse picks her up. Once she has lifted her out of the incubator, she pauses and carefully checks all her wires and tubes to make sure none are dislodged or tangled. Sophie is, after all, still connected to an NG feeding tube, the high-flow oxygen and her monitor checking her breathing rate, heart rate and oxygen saturation. She also has cannulas in both hands delivering fluids and medication and allowing the doctors to take blood samples.

Once the nurse is happy that everything is in order, she places her gently in my arms. Oh, heaven! After everything we've been through since she was born, we have finally reached the moment we have dreamt of but feared would never come. I'm able to hold my baby. Yes, she is covered in wires and, yes, I needed a nurse to get her out of her incubator for me. Nonetheless, it's perfect!

I'm worried about accidentally pulling on one of the wires and hurting or destabilising her but the nurse is very reassuring and checks for me that they are all safe. I ask her whether Sophie will be cold. I'm worried she will get chilly out of her incubator because she is, still, naked except for a nappy. The nurse kindly finds me a blanket to wrap her in as I hold her.

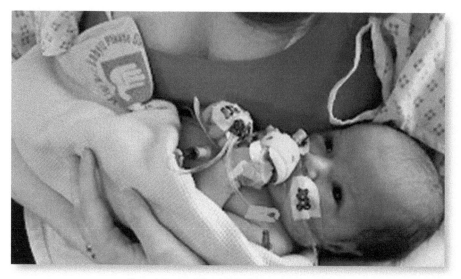

Emma's first cuddle with Sophie at nine days old

Jamie's first cuddle with Sophie

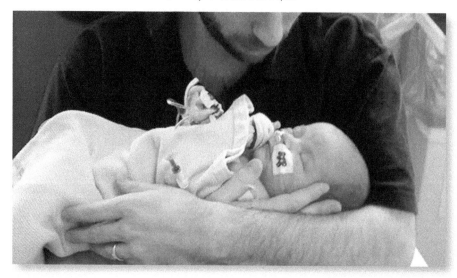

I kiss her little forehead as Jamie takes photos of these precious first cuddles. Cuddles that should have taken place a week earlier but which are even more special because we've had to wait for them. Because they have been promised for so long but so nearly taken away, I never want to put her down. I want to hold her forever and never let her go. I feel she needs to make up for a week's worth of missed cuddles.

◊

I spent most of the rest of Sophie's babyhood cuddling her. I let her nap in my arms after feeds, I carried her around with me as I did housework, I breastfed her until she turned one. I just knew how precious she was and how fortunate we were to be able to hold her at all. I didn't want to do anything else.

Now, I'm so glad I did that. It was terrible for her sleep training but it was so important. I felt I had the chance to make up for everything she'd missed out on in her first days. And it has meant that we are extremely close. It is a cliché, but it is true that small children grow up unbelievably fast. I'm glad I didn't waste a single moment of her babyhood. It flew past and is now a distant memory, but I know that I spent every single moment of it with her, and much of it cuddling her. I didn't miss a second of that brief but special time. It breaks my heart to think of her growing up. That she won't always be a cuddly little girl. But it's extremely comforting to know that I made the most of her infancy.

Since the day Sophie was born, Mum had been sending daily emails to a group of friends and relatives who had asked to be kept up to date. On this day, Mum sent her final update with a picture of me holding Sophie. She sent me an email that evening which just said:

'The whole of Kent is in tears!'

While this was obviously an exaggeration, I was so touched to know that so many people had been following her progress, rooting for her, and thinking of us. Over the preceding days, my entire world had shrunk into Room One and I had lost touch with the outside world. This helped me to reconnect with it, as did the absurd number of cards and presents Sophie received.

February Nineteen

*I*t's my birthday and I receive the best birthday present I could possibly have wished for. Sophie has had such a good night off the ventilator that she's being moved out of intensive care and into high dependency.

This is a whole new world. She's in a cot rather than an incubator, albeit a plastic hospital cot. She's allowed clothes for the first time in her life. And we are able to take a much more active role in looking after her. We're able to pick her up and hold her whenever we want to, we can dress her and change her nappy. We can give her her tube feeds. We can be parents to her.

She's still being tube fed and is still receiving oxygen, but otherwise her life is more or less like that of a healthy baby. She has to finish her course of antibiotics but these are the only medications she's still on.

The downside to being off the medication is that she's addicted to the morphine and has, effectively, to go cold turkey. As a result, for a few days she's very grumpy and agitated. Her pupils are huge and her eyes wide. It's distressing to see. She's so agitated that the doctors have to give her oral tranquilisers to settle her.

Jamie jokes: 'At least we've got drug addiction out of the way early!'

◊

We hadn't yet registered Sophie's birth. Partly because we couldn't think of a suitable middle name. Partly because we were scared. It felt like tempting fate. Like jinxing her somehow. Registering her birth was like certifying that she was a real, new person with a life ahead of her. While she was in intensive care, we didn't feel ready to do that. I think we almost felt like we hadn't earnt the right to do so.

So, once she was safely installed in high dependency, I caught a cab to the registry office in Camden and registered her. It felt like a victory parade. We'd gone through so much to get to this point of certifying her as a permanent new being. I was walking on air. Slightly hyperactive. The official who filled out the birth certificate must have been baffled. She must be used to seeing exhausted new parents regarding this part of having a baby as a chore, so my delight at being there must have been unusual.

I enjoyed quizzing her about some of the oddest names she had registered. I remember double and triple checking that I'd spelt everything right on the form. I knew I'd never live it down if I spelt her name wrong.

When I returned to the hospital Dad was there. My retired lawyer father. As I knew he would, he asked to see the birth certificate. The lawyer in him just can't resist checking official documents for inaccuracies, however slight. I handed it over assertively, glad I had checked it so carefully, but still slightly worried he'd point out a glaring error. I was like a child handing their teacher an essay they had worked hard on and were proud of. Mercifully, Dad gave it the all clear.

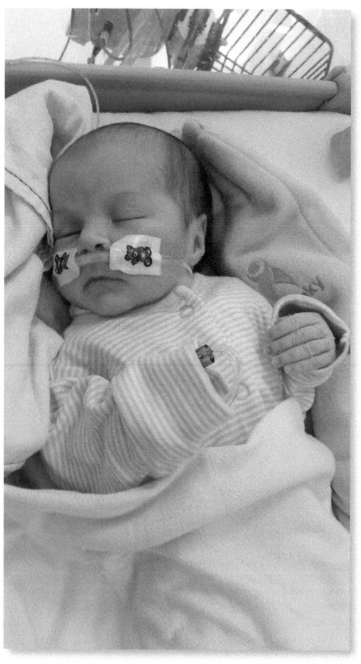

*Sophie's first day in high dependency. Also, her first
day in clothes and without a ventilator!*

Special Care

Sophie spent two nights in high dependency being weaned off the last of her breathing support. Then she was moved further along The Corridor to special care where she spent about a week finishing her antibiotics and practising feeding.

We were so lucky that she came off oxygen so quickly. The doctors initially thought she might need it for months. There had been a suggestion that she might need to go home on oxygen. I saw plenty of parents on the unit being taught how to cope with a baby who was being discharged on oxygen. That could very easily have been us. It was pure good fortune that once she had turned the vital corner, she recovered completely so quickly.

On Sophie's last day in high dependency Jamie wrote in his diary:

> 'I'm fabulous. I'm adorable and have a sweet little face, cute little eyes and the most endearing hiccups.'

Once she was free of all technology, other than her NG feeding tube, we could see her gorgeous little face properly. We could pick her up, cuddle her and change

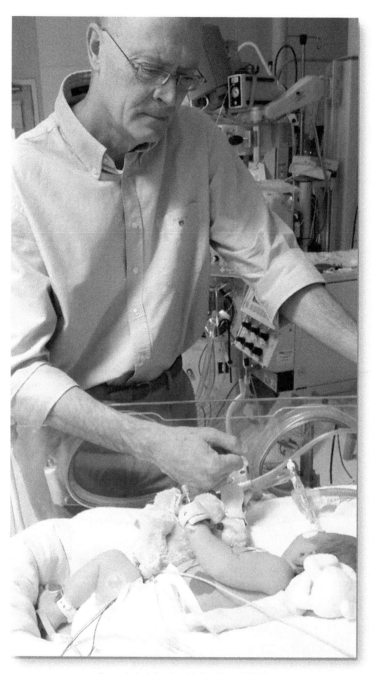

Emma's dad, Paul, with Sophie in NICU

her nappy without worrying about wires and monitors. We could look after her like all other parents look after their newborns.

She seemed to have hiccups most of the time, apparently caused by being overstimulated by the hospital environment. She needed the calm and quiet of our home, not the busy, bright, noisy NICU. It was too much for her newborn, still recovering, body.

In special care there's only one nurse to every four babies so parents are expected to take an active role in caring for their baby. It's a completely different environment to intensive care where the nurses carry out all of the basic care, from giving tube feeds to changing nappies.

We were delighted to be able to look after Sophie ourselves. It felt right. We were finally able to be parents to her. However, once she was awake, fully conscious, and capable of all the same needs, desires and emotions as other newborns, it was much harder leaving her at night. When she was sedated in intensive care, we knew there was nothing we could do for her that the nurses weren't already doing. We knew she probably wasn't even aware we were there. As a result, we didn't feel bad leaving her. In special care it was completely different. We felt guilty. But there was no choice because there was nowhere for us to sleep on the unit. The staff probably would eventually have sent us home to rest, for our own good, if we hadn't gone of our own accord.

We knew that the nurse looking after Sophie would do everything she possibly could for her. All of the nurses were so kind and gentle and attentive. We even knew

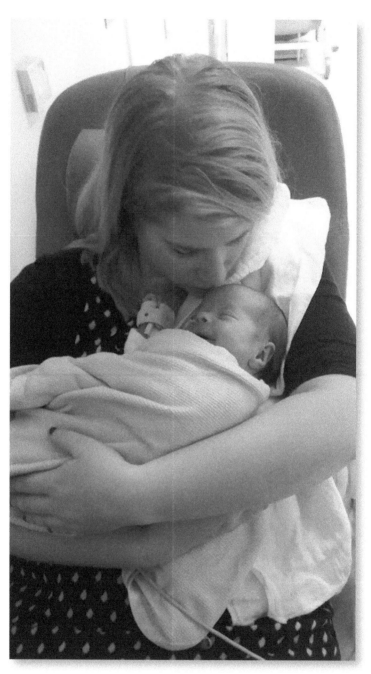

Jamie's sister, Natalie, holding Sophie

that the nurse would cuddle her, assuming she had time. However, we worried that when the nurse was busy tending to another baby Sophie might be left to cry in the night. That she wasn't being held for hours at a time like she would be at home but, rather, that she was spending almost all of the time we weren't there stuck in her cot.

That felt wrong and unnatural. We wanted her home with us as soon as possible so that she could start to receive the round-the-clock, loving, parental care that she needed.

◊

I still find it difficult to think about those nights. When I met one of the consultants years later at a fundraising event, she reassured me that she always tries to pick up any baby that's crying in the night. It's clearly not the same though, as spending hours lying asleep in a parent's arms as they watch TV or a read a book in the evenings.

Each day Sophie was in special care was much like every other so it's hard to remember what happened on individual days. Our time was spent learning how to change nappies, how to give tube feeds and how to comfort a crying baby. We'd never done any of these things before and we had to learn, just as all new parents do. We were lucky, in a way, that we had a team of wonderful nurses to support and teach us. To learn from. To answer our many questions.

I remember panicking on one occasion that Sophie was having a fit because she was squeaking in her sleep and her eyes were rolling back in her head. I was extremely glad that the nurse was there to reassure me that it was completely normal in a newborn. It meant that when we got home and she did it again I knew not to worry.

I was still spending a lot of time in The Dairy as Sophie was getting most of her milk through her tube, but I also received help from the Speech and Language Therapists with establishing breastfeeding. They came to see me every day in a bid to get Sophie exclusively breastfed as quickly as possible, as this was a key requirement before she could be discharged.

While she was in special care, there was frequent talk of moving her to a different hospital. She no longer needed to be at UCLH. Technically, she should have been at our local hospital once she was out of high dependency but each time they tried to transfer her it was full. So we remained at UCLH slightly longer than we might have done. But we were glad of that. It was further for us to travel but we had got to know the unit and the staff and we trusted them and felt safe there.

◊

Finally, when she was eighteen days old, she left UCLH and was transferred back to the Royal Free. A neonatal transfer ambulance arrived and she was strapped into a mobile cot that looked a little like a space capsule.

Thinking about it now, it seems as if for her first few days on earth Sophie was constantly surrounded by dauntingly unfamiliar medical paraphernalia. No wonder, then, that homely objects like Blue Cow were so important to us. I also realise now how wise it was that the NICU gave all babies in its care what are called Zaky Hugs. These life-size beanbags mimic a parent's forearm and hand and are positioned around babies to make them feel as though they are being held.

Sophie still has hers in her bed. She calls it her 'Mummy Hand'.

I asked her recently about this beanbag. She said: 'I love my Mummy Hand because it keeps me safe. I like cuddling it in bed because it is like cuddling your real arm. I can cuddle it in the night when your real arm isn't there.'

Ordinarily, either Jamie or I would have been able to accompany Sophie in the ambulance but the passenger seat was broken so we followed in a taxi. We were pleased to be heading closer to home. It would be much easier having Sophie just a few minutes' walk from our flat, although we had no idea how long she would be there. It could be weeks.

When we arrived, Sophie was being settled in a corner of the Special Care Unit. It was something of a shock after UCLH. It was practically deserted. No other babies or parents were visible and there were barely any staff. Having become accustomed to the busy, reassuringly active, UCLH environment, this was scary.

We felt as if we were being ditched in an abandoned hospital wing. There was no obvious sign of friendly

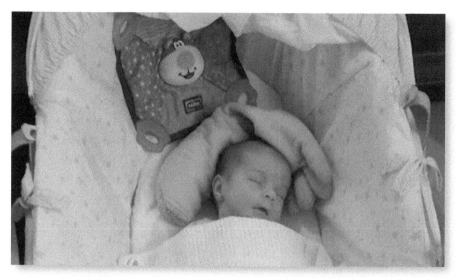

Sophie in her Moses basket with her Zaky Hug the day she left hospital

Sophie on her way from UCLH back to the Royal Free

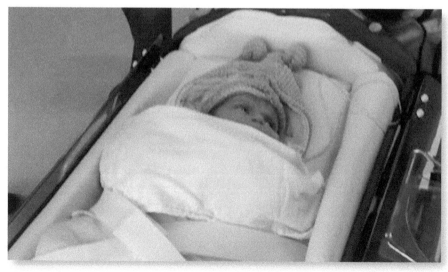

nurses or caring doctors. It also made it a little hard to understand why we had repeatedly been told they were full. We began slightly to wonder whether the truth was that they had avoided taking us in. I'm not sure Sophie's birth had left the staff with happy memories. Maybe they were worried that we would bear them ill-will? This was, after all, where she had become so sick. As it was, we didn't. I have never felt any anger about what happened. I don't have any negative feelings about the care we received and I don't blame anyone. In fact, I feel nothing but gratitude for the care Sophie received and for how lucky we are that she pulled through.

We were initially told that because she was new to the unit Sophie would have to be quarantined in a closed incubator to ensure she didn't bring in any infections. Having got used to her being in a normal cot, this felt like a step backward. When I saw the set up, I cried. I had thought this move would mean getting a step closer to normality – to home. Quite the opposite.

However, just as we were despairing, a caring doctor arrived to welcome us. She said she wasn't concerned about infection and that there was no need for Sophie to be in an incubator after all. She said she could see no reason why she needed to be there, in fact, there was no need for her to be in the nursery at all. Much to our surprise, Sophie was allowed to be in a private 'rooming in' room with us.

They wanted to get her home as quickly as possible and 'rooming in' was the next step. In other words, we would stay with her in a private room, rather like a very nasty hotel room. We would be entirely responsible for her care but there would be nurses outside to help us if we had any concerns and who would check on us periodically.

The doctor also said that Sophie would never learn to breastfeed while she was being given tube feeds – there was no motivation. So, she removed the tube there and then and said she was now to be exclusively breastfed. She told us that Sophie would be discharged as soon as she started to gain weight.

Having expected Sophie to be in a nursery, as she had been at UCLH, this was a bit of a shock. It also came with practical considerations. Now that we were in sole charge of her, one of us had to be in the room with her at all times. We hadn't expected this and didn't have any spare clothes or overnight things with us.

It was also worrying that we no longer had the option of giving top-ups of milk through her NG tube. That had been reassuring while she was learning to feed. I was scared that she might lose more weight or become dehydrated. However, I did agree with the doctor that removing the tube was likely to speed up the process of teaching her to feed properly.

It was very frustrating being stuck in one tiny, hospital room all day. I was able to be with my baby but I had lost my freedom entirely. It would have been alright if, like most parents in these rooms, I'd just given birth and needed to lie in a hospital bed recovering. But Sophie was now three weeks old. I'd completed the most difficult phase of my recovery and was ready to be taking her for walks and going out for coffee with my

NCT friends. Being stuck in this room made me feel like screaming.

While it was difficult being trapped in that room, it was reassuring having nurses just outside to answer our questions. We'd become institutionalised and were used to having a bank of monitors to reassure us that Sophie was okay. We'd also learnt to worry about her breathing rate and her oxygen saturation. As a result, we needed the nurses' reassurances. We needed them to teach us that Sophie was now a healthy baby and that she should be treated as such. We needed to stop viewing her as an intensive care patient and start viewing her as 'normal'. It was a difficult transition to make.

It was hard, too, to get into that mindset because there were hurdles to be crossed before we could be discharged. For example, we were required to attend a first aid session on how to deal with respiratory arrest in a newborn, a training that parents of healthy babies are not required to attend.

It was a private session, given to us by a nurse on night shifts. So training began at ten in the evening! It was stressful and upsetting to be in a tiny side room off the Special Care Unit, late in the evening, being shown how to resuscitate a plastic baby. We were grateful for the training but it hardly felt like a return to normality and it wasn't entirely reassuring that this training was deemed necessary. I had Sophie in a mobile cot next to me during the lesson and I remember that I kept glancing at her to check she was still breathing.

◊

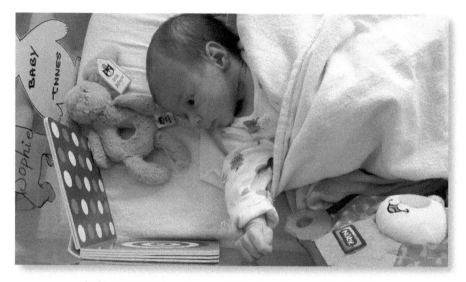

Sophie, completely free of wires and tubes, 'rooming in' at the Royal Free

Sophie on her way home from the Royal Free in the pushchair

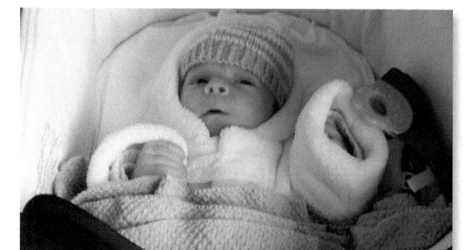

By the time Sophie was twenty days old, and we had spent two nights 'rooming in', she'd put on two grams. Finally, I could push her home in the pushchair. I'd had to wait a lot longer than I'd expected but we'd got there in the end. Jamie had gone back to work so it was Mum who came to help me take Sophie, and our bags, home from the hospital.

We walked out of the hospital and home through Belsize Park, checking on her constantly. I remember half feeling like running home and never going near a hospital again, and half wanting to turn around and take her straight back into their care.

It was a truly special moment when Jamie returned from work that evening to find his little girl finally at home. It had happened three weeks later than it should have done but, at last, she was where she belonged: on the sofa being cuddled by her parents.

◊

Leaving hospital was bittersweet. We were so happy to be able to take Sophie home. To have her with us and not to have to keep traipsing up and down to the hospital. But the UCLH NICU had also become a second home. We'd got to know the staff, other parents and the routine. On some level, we had become institutionalised and our connection to the place ran deep. We were sad to leave. We knew that we would immediately be replaced by another family in need of help and that life on the unit would continue without us. It didn't need us. But we would always feel a deep bond with it, despite having been there for less than three weeks. There was a feeling of loss leaving the safety of that institution. Similar to the feeling of leaving a school you've been happy at.

Initially, I was terrified. It was scary not having the monitors to reassure me that Sophie was fine. I'd got used to having kind, experienced nurses to help me and to answer my string of questions. I missed that and felt vulnerable without them. Looking after her by myself when Jamie went back to work was particularly unnerving.

She was so very young and still recovering from her illness and her treatment. As a result, she slept almost constantly during her first few weeks at home. She wouldn't wake up for feeds. Left to her own devices, she would have slept for twelve or fourteen hours straight, without feeding. She had become used to having milk poured down her tube as she slept – she hadn't learnt to wake up when she needed milk. This makes her sound like a dream baby. But it wasn't like that. It was extremely stressful because she still weighed less than she had at birth and she wasn't gaining weight. She needed regular feeds. We ended up spending hours trying to wake her up to feed. But she wouldn't stir. We tried taking her outside in the cold, changing her nappy; we tried talking to her. We tried everything we could think of to wake her up and feed her. But all she wanted to do was sleep.

A few days after she had left hospital, I started to panic because she had been asleep for fourteen hours. In the end, in tears, I took her to paediatric A&E at our local hospital. I told the triage nurse all about it. Needless to say, she was rushed straight through and seen immediately by the paediatricians. Of course, as soon as they walked in, she woke up and started vocally demanding milk. It was embarrassing but they were extremely sympathetic and reassuring, saying how delighted they were to see that she was now awake and feeding. They were very understanding about our situation and could see how scared and worried I was. Many of them had been involved in her care immediately after her birth so they understood what we'd been through.

They told me not to worry about waking her up – just to let her sleep as sleep was what she needed. They helped me to understand exactly how much milk she needed and when I should worry. They were very helpful and, after that, I was less stressed about her feeding.

Over time, I relaxed. She was gaining weight, growing, smiling and becoming more alert. I began to enjoy motherhood and my baby without constantly fearing for her safety.

◊

Until Sophie was one, she was seen regularly by the paediatricians at the Royal Free. She also had very detailed developmental follow-up at the hospital until she turned two. This was mainly to monitor her for any signs of brain damage. It was also because she was part of a research study into the effects of cooling. Each appointment, particularly the developmental ones, was fraught with anxiety for us. We could see that she appeared to be doing well, but we were still scared that the tests would flag up a problem. I both dreaded and looked forward to these appointments. I dreaded them because I was scared of the results, but also cautiously looked forward to them because I hoped they would give me reassurance. A large part of me knew that she was fine, but I still needed that reassurance.

The developmental assessments were extremely detailed. At each one, the doctor would assess Sophie's fine and gross motor skills, her language and communication skills and her social skills. I was always fascinated to see what tests she was required to pass. They seemed so random but I understood that there was solid science behind them. Did she hold her feet when she was lying on the floor? Did she throw a rubber duck she was given across the room? Did she hold a piece of paper still with one hand while drawing with the other?

We were extremely fortunate – miraculously so. No problems were ever discovered at the paediatric appointments or at the developmental ones. As a result, when she turned two, she was discharged from all follow-up care. It was the official end of the medical journey that had begun the day she was born.

At one of the appointments, I asked the doctor whether it was possible to have HIE Grade Two and not to have any problems as a result. She shrugged in Sophie's direction and said: 'Seemingly so.'

I asked: 'How do you know? How can you say that without examining her?'

The doctor replied, 'I believe that you can tell if a baby is healthy by whether you smile when you look at them. Looking at her puts a huge grin on my face.'

Part Three
Reflections

Jamie's Reflections

Kindness and Florentines

It's often said that you learn the most about yourself during your toughest times. I would say Sophie's illness taught me more about other people. About how good and kind they are, even to those they have never met.

The care we received from the medical staff, and the love from our family, were so valuable to us. The attentiveness of the nurses. The cool calm of the doctors. The look of love in my mother's eyes. Her warm, comforting words. I cannot remember what they were but they were just what I needed to hear at the time. The creativity of my sister, determined to challenge the sense of dread hanging over us. The calm reassurance of Emma's father, Paul. The pragmatic care from her mother, Caroline. All of infinite importance and so beyond words. Perhaps all of the most important feelings, interactions and moments with others are beyond words because they happen in the eyes, as much as in the deed. It's the look and the tone. The soft touch. These are the true foundations for the majesty of humanity.

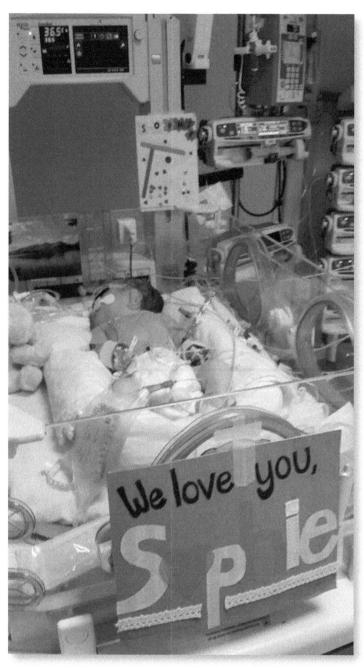

Natalie's sign at the end of Sophie's incubator in NICU

But it wasn't just the medics and our families. Many people touched our lives during this time. People we might not have expected to, and often in practical but equally significant ways. Here are some of those kindnesses in no particular order:

At the beginning of our time in the NICU Sophie was in purgatory. Between life and death. In a clinical cot where life is not really life. Between identity and non-identity. When we decided on Sophie as a name, Natalie made a beautiful pink card with 'Sophie' written across the front. It was stuck at the end of her cot and brought the only source of colour to an otherwise sterile intensive care bed. It gave us hope, and perhaps it even helped Sophie seem like a person, even though she was sedated and covered in wires. No one asked Natalie to do this. It just came to her, as kind gestures so often do in her case. It made all the difference to Sophie's corner of Room One.

◊

A friend of ours, Laura, stitched together a beautiful handmade quilt for Sophie. It has white, pink and blue patches with a blue border and a light floral pattern. It's soft but feels resilient. Sophie's initials, SEI, are in the corner. It has a lovely, homely, safe feel. It arrived one day without any fanfare. What a precious expression of skill and love. What could be more comforting or homely than a quilt? It sits today as a throw over Sophie's reading chair. She loves doing arts and crafts so maybe one day she will make one for someone else; will pass on the gesture that meant so much to us.

◊

When Sophie was born normal life stopped. I messaged work the day after her birth to explain the situation in brief. The school where I then worked was very supportive – the Headmaster told me quite strictly that I was not to worry about work or pay cheques, but to take time to look after my family.

I later learnt that friends in my department, Matt and Rob, had started to get suspicious that they'd not heard from me following my departure from school when Emma went into labour. The Senior Master, Tim, had obviously kept my situation quiet, so no one knew what had happened, and I wasn't in the right state of mind even to think of messaging. But, apparently during a lunch break, Matt had collared Tim in the corridor to find out what had happened to me.

It amuses me to imagine this scene: a pugnacious free-speaking Northerner ambushing an old school, southern, public school master who also happens to look like Bill Clinton.

It meant a lot that they cared. Matt came to visit me once or twice in central London. His calm, practical, honest yet positive, no-nonsense self was a great tonic, especially during the period when we didn't know if Sophie would live, or if she would be able to live 'normally' following the oxygen starvation. Some people are good friends. Some people become good friends when things get tough.

◊

One of Emma's mother's friends from Kent, Carolyne, sent us home-made florentines. The proof of how beautifully they were made was that we found them exquisite even though we had lost virtually all interest in food. Who would have thought chocolate, caramelised almonds, soft fruit, and a bit of unexpected care from someone I didn't even know would be such an effective antidote to the dark thoughts that occupied us during so many troubled evenings?

◊

When I'm stressed and scared, I often look for ways to control events around me in order to feel I have more agency. A flaw perhaps, but a natural one, my inclination was to try to understand the science and the medicine behind Sophie's conditions and her treatment. This was partly to make sense of what was unfolding and partly because the instinct to protect my child was so strong that I wanted to be as capable as possible of contributing to her care. Obviously I could make no real difference but it was important for me to try.

Enter my personal hero in this story, Dr Giles Kendall. Dr Kendall has enormous intelligence, an ebullient curiosity and a wonderful drive to educate. Each time he came to see Sophie on his ward rounds he took the time to define key terms, explain what the different processes were and how they applied to Sophie. This was a kindness because Dr Kendall was always busier than it's possible to be, but he still found the time and energy to speak to me. However, he also seemed excited that, finally, there was a parent who was actually interested in understanding persistent pulmonary hypertension and

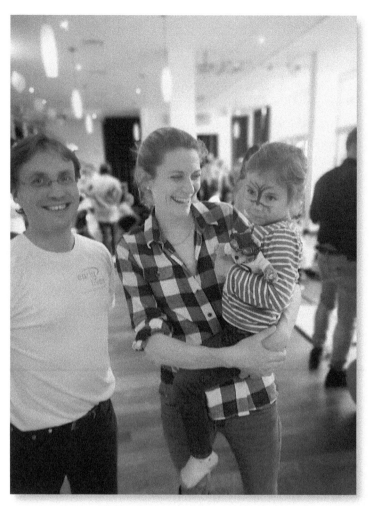

A shy Sophie, and Emma, with Dr Kendall at a party
for NICU graduates in November 2019

the resulting shunting in the circulatory system. For me, it meant empowerment. It was a way to move beyond being a helpless victim – and it was very interesting.

I remember two distinct examples of his kindness. The first was when he came over with a piece of paper, drew a schematic diagram of the circulatory system, and explained how different drugs and kit were being deployed to overcome an issue that was causing Sophie's oxygen saturation to drop. Compassion. Love of learning. Love of teaching. Values that, as a teacher myself, are very important to me. It didn't change the fact that Sophie was sick. But it meant that when there was finally progress, I understood the significance of her blood pressure normalising, the significance of nitrogen being removed, the significance of the doctors lowering the frequency of the oscillator.

The second was towards the end of Sophie's time in intensive care, when she went for an MRI scan to examine, among other things, the damage to her brain. As the initial cold terror of losing Sophie subsided, it was replaced with a nagging anxiety that all might not be well in the future. Was her brain irreparably damaged? Dr Kendall came to see me in person to show me the results. Brain imaging and the clever electro-microscopy that goes with it are two of his fields of specialism. He so generously took time out of his busy schedule to show me a few graphs (I couldn't help noticing the impish grin on his face). He had put them together to provide me with scientific evidence of Sophie's brain health. Then those precious words: 'She's well below the bottom end of the range. There's a vanishingly small chance of brain damage.' I couldn't really believe in that random graph on the page in the same way he could. But it seems he was right. The fact that he came to see me and to explain what it meant as one adult to another meant so much to me.

◊

Professor Wyatt was another of my heroes. When he heard about our situation from Natalie, he was immediately kind and supportive. Would we like to speak to him? It would be no problem. I remember a phone call. A bit of parental counselling/therapy and some expert advice. He had a warm, trustworthy and reassuring voice. He talked us through the situation. He didn't sugar-coat it but we felt better for it. Then he offered to come in to visit. We were staggered. Wasn't he retired? Whatever, it felt right. So, yes please!

Where do these heroes get their energy from? Was Professor Wyatt's visit a turning point, another guardian angel? He certainly offered invaluable advice about Sophie's care. He didn't need to come, but he came because he cared about a stranger's baby.

◊

On The NHS

I don't remember our local hospital very happily, given what happened there. However, the medical staff were hit with a very unusual and critical emergency which they were not well-resourced to deal with.

There's no doubt that without the rapid and effective care they gave Sophie once she was delivered, she would have died very quickly. While we didn't get to know these doctors as we did the ones at UCLH, they were equally critical in saving Sophie's life.

All the staff in the UCLH NICU are heroes. We owe them Sophie's life, and all our happiness for the boundless gifts Sophie has brought us. They saved us from all the unhappiness of the void that would have opened up before us had we lost her.

The NHS isn't perfect, but we are immensely grateful for it. I no longer mind paying my taxes as long as I imagine they are going to the NICU. Boris Johnson is an unlikely source to quote at this stage, but when he said that the NHS is unstoppable because it is 'powered by love' I felt he had got it about right.[4] We owe so much love to the NHS.

◊

On Sophie

And to Sophie. To me Sophie is perfection. Sophie is worthy of absolute love. I love her ad absurdum. I understand this love all the more because I know how close it was to never being. Because she was so close to dying before she was even known.

'Run faster Daddy! We are nearly where the naughty sheep have escaped in my school field.'

Sophie is wearing a grey Gap hoodie with pink writing. She has on leggings and her running shoes. She is pulling me along the pavement of a park in Tonbridge. This is her third Park Run. On her first she did the two-kilometre course in more than twenty minutes with many breaks and much encouragement.

She's made so much progress. 'Don't go through the funnel with me Daddy', she says as we near the finish. Like her mother, she is a stickler for the rules and loves reminding me of my responsibilities. When she crosses the line, she says 'thank you' to the staff in her beautiful, slightly lispy way. She's done it in under sixteen minutes. We go to the playground to celebrate.

'I love Park Run Daddy.'

She's not always enthusiastic and has the same capacity as any child to be grumpy and uninterested. But fundamentally she has such enthusiasm and is refreshingly free-spirited. These qualities are epitomised in the sweetest little phrases or with a tone of voice which so freely and generously gives significance to even the smallest of moments. This moment was special to me. For someone who came so close to death due to lung damage to be completing a two-kilometre run in style. What a little hero!

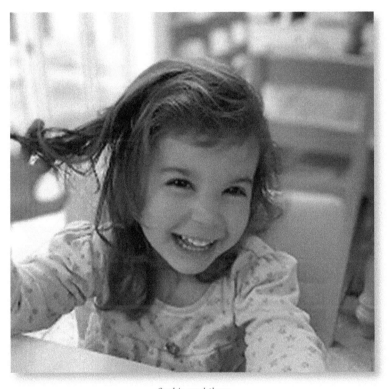

Sophie aged three

Emma's Reflections

Sophie is now four and she is heaven. She and her little brother George are everything to us. The smell of their soft skin, the warmth of their little bodies, the gentleness of their nature ... They are perfect to me and I adore them.

My godmother said she thought Sophie's birth had 'blown my heart wide open'. She was right. Sophie made me more emotionally open and sensitive and that was the best present anyone has ever given me. She and George are the most precious gifts I've ever received. They have made me a better person, have made my life – my happiness – inextricably bound up with other people. With that comes vulnerability and the end of self-sufficiency; it also brings huge joy and meaning.

The children have taught me that to experience the greatest love and joy you also have to allow that fragility into your life. They have taught me so much: gentleness and compassion, the power of maternal love and the importance of having someone to cherish. Sophie showed us that as long as everyone we hold dear is safe, nothing else really matters.

Sophie is sweet and kind and calm. Polite and funny and cheeky. She wants to please and doesn't like being in trouble. She also has a mischievous streak (inherited from her father) and loves a challenge.

She loves playing with her little brother, cuddling her puppy and cooking. She enjoys gymnastics, arts and crafts and flying around on her scooter.

Every day I look at her and I feel just so lucky to have her. I don't know why she got so sick nor do I know why she survived. I feel unworthy of such good fortune. This story could so very easily have had a different ending.

At Christmas, I watched her as a donkey in her first Nativity play. Wearing big donkey ears this little three-year-old introduced the whole performance to the watching parents. Tears streamed down my face. How lucky we are to have her and how amazing it is that she is so perfect. How can a woman's body create something so wonderful? How can medical science, and the miracle workers who practise it, have preserved such perfection in such dire straits?

Her milestones will always come with an extra dose of emotion for me, because we so nearly didn't get to witness them. I spent ten days sitting beside her as she fought for her life in intensive care. I listened to doctors explaining that she was probably going to die. I lay in bed at night wondering whether I was about to plan her funeral. I lived in fear of my phone ringing in the middle of the night to tell me she had died. Those experiences will always be with me.

Every night, when I put her to bed, I give her an extra kiss. Because I can. Each morning when I drop her at school, I give her an extra cuddle. In the afternoons my heart sings as I walk to collect her, because soon she'll be back by my side.

◊

For Sophie's sake I wish none of this had ever happened. I wish that I had had an uneventful caesarean on the due date and that she had been born alert, kicking and screaming. It would, undeniably, have been better for her if she had received the skin-to-skin contact and breastfeeding newborns so desperately need.

It's unnerving to think of the impact on her little body of having been so unwell, and of receiving such aggressive treatment. Because surely that has to leave a legacy within the body? So far, she appears to have escaped completely unscathed; seems to be absolutely fine. But I retain a nagging doubt. A fear that at some point a legacy from the experience will become apparent.

So, without a doubt, if I could go back in time, I would do everything possible to protect her, to save her from that experience. For her sake.

As for Jamie and me, I'm not so sure. We tasted hell; we travelled a long way down the road to purgatory; we stared death in the face. We were presented with the very real prospect of losing our daughter – surely the worst thing a parent can face.

It has undoubtedly left us both with scars. But I don't know if I would choose for it not to have happened. We emerged from the experience and I think we emerged as better and wiser people. The most intense experience of our lives and, surely, as Jamie reflected earlier, powerful experiences are what life is all about. A life without them may be comfortable and easy but slightly empty? Shallow, maybe.

◊

Before Sophie was born, we knew we wanted to have more than one child, wanted her to have a playmate, a companion close to her in age. However, after her birth, the concept of having another baby took on a whole new meaning. For months I couldn't even begin to face the idea.

But, when Sophie was about eighteen months old, we started trying for another baby. First time round, it had been exciting. An adventure. This time it was scary and daunting. We knew what we were getting into.

I got pregnant very quickly. When I found out I was pregnant with Sophie, I sat Jamie down, gave him a cuddle and told him in an excited and loving way. This time, I called Jamie while he was at work.

'What's up?' He asked. 'Is everything okay? I'm busy and stressed!'

I said: 'I think I'm about to make you more stressed but, hopefully, in a good way …'

'Oh God! You're pregnant!'

◊

During the pregnancy we agonised over the best delivery option. What would be safest for our second child? I spoke to the consultants looking after me during this pregnancy and had a meeting with the consultant who had investigated what went wrong during Sophie's birth.

It was difficult. No one really knew why Sophie was so unwell when she was born and, as a result, no one could be certain they could stop it happening again. All the doctors I spoke to said that, theoretically, it should be safe for me to have another natural delivery. They said I would be on Labour Ward with continuous monitoring. That, this time, I would be given antibiotics during the labour to reduce the risk of infection and that they would intervene to deliver the baby if there was even a hint that he was struggling.

Even with all this reassurance, I was still nervous.

As a result, I eventually requested a planned caesarean. When pushed on the topic, the consultant agreed it was probably the safer option. I was acutely aware of my obligation to Sophie – I knew that my safety mattered because she needed me. However, I couldn't put another baby in danger. Couldn't risk him going through the same experience as Sophie.

For a week before the caesarean, I burst into tears every time I looked at Sophie. My perception of the risks involved in childbirth had become so skewed that I was convinced I would die on the operating table and leave her alone, without a mother.

As it turned out, I needn't have been so scared. It was an intense and frightening experience but, unlike the natural delivery, it felt like a controlled situation. The surgery was quick and straightforward and, thankfully, George was delivered, weighing seven pounds twelve. Jamie and I both cried when we heard him scream moments after he was born.

I lay in recovery after the operation and couldn't believe I had him with me and that he was safe. The relief was overwhelming. That he was out and we were both okay. I felt so lucky to have a healthy baby in my arms. A baby attached to no wires or machines. A baby who wasn't about to be whisked away by medics. Finally, we were experiencing childbirth as it's meant to be.

The day after George was born, I was discharged from hospital and arrived home at Sophie's bedtime. She wanted to cuddle her new brother so I tucked him up in bed next to her for a moment so she could see him and give him a hug. For a moment it looked as if he was smiling, warm and cosy lying there next to his sister.

I think that was the happiest moment of my life.

As I write this, George is about to turn two and he is lying in my arms in his sleeping bag having somehow dodged going to bed. A healthy little boy who was spared the traumas his sister experienced.

George has made our family complete. He has tousled blonde hair and big blue eyes. He has the cheekiest, most mischievous little face with a naughty grin and a twinkle in his eye. He loves tractors and racing cars

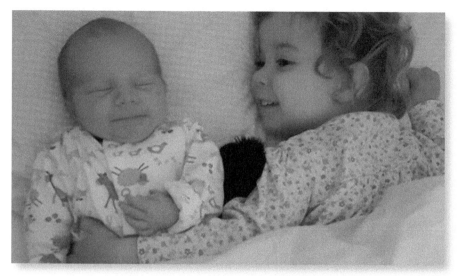

Sophie cuddling George the day after he was born in June 2018

George

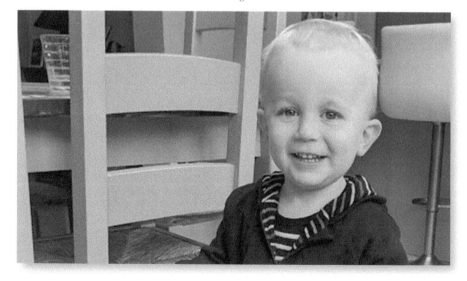

and aeroplanes. He likes throwing stones and getting soaking wet jumping in puddles. He doesn't believe any space on his plate should be wasted on vegetables and shouts: 'No! It's horrible! Take vegetables away!'

He's also cuddly and affectionate and sweet. He says to me, Jamie, Sophie, and even the dog, numerous times a day: 'I love you, whole world!' He is often to be found balancing precariously on Sophie's window ledge having climbed on to it to look for the neighbour's cat over the garden fence. Then he says, 'Georgie want kitten too! A pink one!'

We are so glad that we braved childbirth again to add him to our family.

◊

Now to the NICU. Here words almost fail me. Sophie is called Sophie Elizabeth after the Elizabeth Garrett Anderson Unit. It seemed apt. We wanted to give her a middle name that had significance. What could possibly be more significant? Without that unit she wouldn't be here today.

It's near impossible to describe the NICU in a way that does it justice. It encapsulates, in one small corridor, both heaven and hell. Many of the experiences there are hellish, but the people who work there are akin to angels trying to save people from hell.

I note that in this book I've used the word kind over thirty times. This is fitting because kindness was at the heart of our experience. Kindness not only from friends and family, but also from strangers.

It's impossible for the parents on the unit to view the staff, the consultants particularly, as anything short of demigods. All of your hopes and fears rest on them – on their skill, knowledge and kindness. You hang on their every word, desperate for them to offer a ray of hope when your baby is clinging to the very fringes of life. They have the power to give you hope or to break your heart forever.

I have often wondered how they cope. How they live that life. How that can be their nine to five. Except that it isn't nine to five. It's eight to eight. More. It isn't a job, surely? It's a way of life, a vocation. They can't just clock off at five in the afternoon, turn their computers off and head to the pub. Can they?

They live with the knowledge that even when they are not in the unit, their colleagues are. Be it Christmas Day, the middle of the night or a Bank Holiday, the work of the unit continues. There are always babies that need them. Always more families depending on them. Always more little lives to be fought for.

Those doctors and nurses, their colleagues see the unimaginable every day. One minute they are discharging a baby who has recovered and can finally go home, the next they're declaring a newborn baby dead. I can't even begin to imagine how they cope. The raw emotions they must witness. The roller coaster of feelings must never leave them. There must be patients, cases, families that haunt them, images they can't escape from.

And yet there they are every day. They keep doing it. They keep going. They keep working with dedication and compassion. Think of the legacy they leave. Without them, thousands of families like ours would be without their precious children. Without them, the promise of new life would result in heartbreak. What they do is truly mind-blowing and we will forever be in awe of them.

This book is written, in large part, as an appreciation of all that they do. In many ways it is also a love story. When Jamie and I met and were enjoying the carefree days of a young romance, we never dreamt what lay ahead. This is true for all of us but perhaps what the experience has most shown us, and we hope you too, is that whatever the outcome, there are always people, often strangers, there to bring light into darkness.

References

1. Great Ormond Street Hospital For Children (2016), *Persistent Pulmonary Hypertension of the Newborn (PPHN)*. Available at https://www.gosh.nhs.uk/conditions-and-treatments/conditions-we-treat/persistent-pulmonary-hypertension-newborn-pphn (Accessed: 18.07.2020)

2. Mosalli, R. (2012) Whole Body Cooling for Infants with Hypoxic-Ischemic Encephalopathy, *Journal of Clinical Neonatology* 2012 Apr-Jun 1 (2): 101–106. doi: 10.4103/2249-4847.96777

3. Yousafzai, Z. (2018) *Let Her Fly: A Father's Journey and the Fight for Equality*. London: WH Allen

4. Johnson, A. [@BorisJohnson] (2020) It is hard to find the words to express my debt to the NHS for saving my life [Twitter] 12 April. Available at: https://twitter.com/BorisJohnson/status/1249336590482243585?s=09

5. Hinton, L. Locock, L. Knight, M. (2014), Partner Experiences of 'NearMiss' Events in Pregnancy and Childbirth in the UK: A Qualitative Study, *PLoS ONE* 9(4): e91735. doi:10.1371/journal.pone.0091735

6. Yousafzai (2018) *Let Her Fly*

Acknowledgements

There are so many people without whom this book would never have come into existence. Much as I would like to thank and acknowledge every single one by name, that simply isn't possible.

First, thank you, with all my heart, to every one of the medics involved in Sophie's care. Every doctor, nurse, physiotherapist, paramedic, pharmacist ... Each of you played a role in saving her life and we couldn't be more grateful. Staff from the Royal Free Hospital, the London NTS and UCLH.

Dr Giles Kendall and Dr Angela Huertas-Ceballos, neonatal consultants at UCLH. This whole book is a tribute to your work, kindness and skill. You gave us hope, made us smile and saved our baby. No words can ever be enough to thank you.

Also, Dr Melanie Menden who cared for Sophie at the Royal Free and Zak Rania, Jerome and Mick from the NTS.

My parents, Caroline and Paul Phippen, Jamie's mum, Mary Embleton, and Jamie's sister, Natalie Tidmarsh, for trekking back and forth to UCLH to be with us while

Sophie was unwell. And for all of your love and support before her birth, and since.

Harriet, Danny and Finn Brennan for allowing us to include their story in this book and for being such wonderful friends ever since we were in the NICU.

Anthea Church (who features in this book as my godmother) for so generously giving her time to edit this book, as well as for supporting and encouraging me and my writing ever since I was at school.

Alison Shakspeare, at Shakspeare Editorial, for her patience, skill and wisdom in editing and formatting this book – I would never have got to this stage without your help. And to Cali Mackrill for designing the book's beautiful cover and for putting up with my endless emails and nitpicking.

All those who kindly agreed to read early drafts of this book and gave invaluable feedback – Keir Hoffman, Frances Hedgeland, Anna Jenkinson and Nell Wyatt.

Hannah Dyesmith and Laura Mackrill for being a huge source of support and friendship to me and Jamie while Sophie was in hospital.

Matt Prestshaw and Rob Simmonds for the compassion you showed Jamie while Sophie was ill.

And, of course, to Jamie for being my rock, my best friend and the best husband and father anyone could wish for.

Emma Innes, September 2022

Lightning Source UK Ltd.
Milton Keynes UK
UKHW020839180123
415542UK00011B/230